Managed Care:

An Occupational Therapy SourceBook

Prepared by
The American Occupational Therapy Association
Managed Care Project Team

▼   Education Department

▼   Ethics Program

▼   Government Relations Department

▼   Practice Department

▼   Public Relations Department

▼   Research, Information, and Evaluation Program

with support from
The American Occupational Therapy Foundation
Wilma L. West Library

We wish to thank the following members from the volunteer sector for their contributions:
Nancy Beck, MA, OTR/L
Thom Fisher, MS, OTR/L, CCM, FAOTA
Maureen Freda, MA, OTR
Sue Harris, OTR
Cynthia Horn-McCoy, OTR
Deborah Williams, OTR

22389

WB
555
.M266
1996

March 1996

American Occupational Therapy Association, Inc.

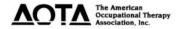

AOTA The American
Occupational Therapy
Association, Inc.

Contents

Managed Care and the Changing Health Care Environment

INTRODUCTION

America's health care system is undergoing rapid change, with individuals increasingly receiving their health care coverage under "managed care," a term used to describe health care systems that integrate the financing and delivery of health services. By combining the traditional roles of both insurance companies in paying for health services and health care providers in overseeing and delivering care, managed care organizations (MCOs) are able to create incentives that channel consumers to selected providers that meet the MCO's quality and cost standards.

The emergence of managed care as the dominant method for controlling health care costs has led to consolidation and integration of health service delivery systems, as hospitals and other providers seek to become more efficient and more cost-effective and to offer a broader array of services. These efforts to become more competitive in the health care marketplace are, in turn, increasing pressures on all health care professionals to redesign their approach to patient care and to more intensively manage clinical resources and demonstrate the effectiveness of their interventions.

Many of the major issues confronting the occupational therapy profession today have their roots in this cost containment imperative and the phenomenon of managed care, ranging from the debate over the appropriate use of noncredentialed personnel to the need for more definitive research demonstrating the efficacy and cost-effectiveness of occupational therapy interventions.

These changes are presenting occupational therapy practitioners—and all health professionals—with major challenges to the traditional philosophical and ethical contexts in which they have been schooled, and they are compelling practitioners to fundamentally reexamine their approach to (clinical) practice in all settings. As AOTA President Mary Foto noted in her presidential address at the Association's 1995 annual conference: to meet the challenge of the changing environment, occupational therapy (OT) practitioners must make

"...changes in our perception of ourselves as well as how we perceive our customers (patients, family, payer) and changes in our patterns of practice."

To effectively make the changes necessary to adapt, occupational therapy practitioners must recognize that the system transformation under way represents a paradigm shift. In the new paradigm, health care is a commodity the purchase of which will increasingly be governed by the rules of the marketplace. Put simply, the provision of occupational therapy or any other health service no longer represents revenue and profit for the facility or provider. Rather, these services now represent a cost that must be effectively managed.

Among the challenges to the profession articulated by AOTA President Foto are

▼ the need to define more clearly the distinctions between treatment—which requires the unique knowledge, skills, and judgment of an OT practitioner—and care—which encompasses services that can be provided by others;

▼ the need for practitioners to recognize they now have dual roles in striving for both clinical excellence and effective resource management; and

▼ the imperative to demonstrate to payers the efficacy, cost-effectiveness, and value that occupational therapy intervention brings to the health care equation.

The opportunities for the profession include a wider role for occupational therapy practitioners in a system that seeks value, and the flexibility to design and provide treatment based on client needs rather than artificial employer or insurance company requirements. Understanding the forces that are propelling these system changes is essential to identifying both internal and external challenges for the occupational therapy profession and the opportunities they present.

BACKGROUND

The way we organize, finance, and deliver health care services in the United States is undergoing profound change. That change is being driven primarily by spending for health care services that has risen much faster than population growth or inflation in the underlying economy.

The rapid increase in health care spending has been fueled by several factors. They include the traditional "fee-for-service" payment methods used by insurers and other third party payers, which encouraged and promoted the provision of more rather than fewer services; and comprehensive health insurance, which has insulated many consumers from an awareness of the actual costs of care. Providers of services have been free to order or provide whatever services they wanted with little concern or accountability for the cost consequences of those decisions. This expansion of the health care sector has also meant more jobs, more opportunities for health care professionals, and more diversity in consumer choice of treatment alternatives and delivery sites.

However, the health care marketplace has now changed direction in important ways. The purchasers of health care—both private (e.g., employers) and public (e.g., government [Medicare, Medicaid])—are determined to become major participants in charting the future direction and control of the health delivery system. These purchasers are now looking at the marketplace for health care from a perspective in which business considerations—most notably cost—are dominant.

This shift in buyer perspective is driving the fundamental changes in the ways in which future services will be delivered. At the core of the purchaser's belief is that consumers and providers must be directly aware of the costs of their decisions about the quantity, type, and site of the health services demanded and delivered. To achieve this objective, purchasers have designed and are implementing payment methods to secure spending control. Responding to this is a whole range of new entities concerned about the financing and/or delivery of care. These include MCOs, integrated provider-based systems such as physician-hospital organizations, utilization information and management firms, quality review companies, and many others—all of whose activities affect the interests of patients and providers alike.

3

HEALTH CARE SPENDING GROWTH

Health care is the largest industry in the United States. Spending for health services grew by more than 250 percent between 1980 and 1993. In 1980, health spending amounted to 9 percent of the nation's total domestic output; by 1993, spending for health accounted for nearly 14 percent. Recent data on health spending provide some indication of a slowdown in the rate of increase in health spending, which (in the minds of some observers) is due to marketplace changes that have had a significant impact on private-sector spending. Public-sector spending for health care, most of which is for the elderly and disabled under Medicare and low-income persons under Medicaid, continues to grow much faster than the private sector.

PRIVATE-SECTOR TRENDS

About 60 percent of the U.S. population have health benefit protection through their employers, while another 6 percent purchase individual coverage. Many employers that provide health coverage are limiting their costs by changing the types of plans they offer, increasing employees' share of the premiums and cost-sharing requirements, or dropping some benefits altogether.

Though many employers still offer some traditional health plan coverage, the number offering some type of managed care coverage is growing dramatically. Well over half of all workers (and their dependents) now have managed care coverage available to them, and even much of the existing traditional indemnity insurance coverage includes elements of managed care. Two of every three employees covered in employer-sponsored plans of employers with more than 500 workers are now enrolled in managed care. Health maintenance organization enrollment, in particular, is growing rapidly.

To control costs, managed care plans use several techniques that limit either provider payments or enrollee use of services. Managed care organizations curb payments through negotiating with providers or through risk-sharing arrangements ("risk sharing" refers to contractual arrangements between MCOs and providers under which set payment amounts are furnished to the provider in exchange for which the provider shares or assumes total responsibility (or risk) for furnishing all or certain health services that a patient may need over a specified period of time).

Such arrangements may restrict an enrollee's choice of provider to those involved in a contractual agreement with the MCO. This type of arrangement usually means lower cost sharing for the enrollees if they obtain care from the providers on the MCO's provider panel(s). Managed care organizations (and most other health plans) also employ utilization review methods to curtail inappropriate service use. They can include preadmission certification, concurrent utilization review, case management programs, and penalties for nonurgent use of the emergency department.

PUBLIC-SECTOR PLANS

Until recently, the major publicly financed health programs—particularly Medicare and Medicaid—have relied on (a) controlling the prices governments are willing to pay (through mechanisms like the Medicare physician fee schedule) and (b) bundling strategies to control costs (through mechanisms like Medicare's Prospective Payment System, which uses diagnosis related groups for hospital reimbursement). Government involvement in managed care has lagged behind developments in the private sector, but that is rapidly changing.

Medicare managed care is just beginning to take on major significance for the future of the program. Until recently, growth in Medicare managed care enrollment was relatively slow for a number of reasons, including inadequate rates paid to managed care organizations.

Enrollment in Medicare managed care has doubled since 1987 and is now growing at double-digit rates—though only 1 of 11 beneficiaries is now enrolled in managed care.

Congress is currently weighing new options to encourage more Medicare beneficiaries to enroll in managed care by making participation in the program more attractive to managed care organizations and by providing new financial and other incentives for the elderly to enroll in such plans. Congress has already approved legislation to expand managed care options (known as Medicare Select plans) for coverage supplementary to the basic Medicare program (traditionally known as Medigap insurance). These efforts are designed to bring the Medicare program more into line with options available in the private sector and to take advantage of managed care's cost-saving techniques to achieve reductions in federal budget expenditures.

State Medicaid programs vary widely in the methods used to purchase care for low-income individuals and families. Recently, many states have adopted new methods for delivering or paying for Medicaid services, including the enrollment of some low-income persons in managed care arrangements. Waivers from existing federal regulations have been granted to numerous states allowing them considerable latitude to develop or experiment with cost-effective alternatives to traditional approaches in their Medicaid programs.

> Much of the reorganization of health care is being prompted by the actions of insurers and managed care organizations.

Managed care is now part of the Medicaid plans in 42 states. About one in every four recipients is in a managed care arrangement—either in primary care case management kinds of programs or in fully capitated programs for certain services. Nevertheless, 93 percent of total Medicaid payments are still made under more traditional fee-for-service arrangements involving the provision of long-term care in nursing facilities rather than acute care services.

PROVIDER RESPONSES TO THE CHANGING MARKETPLACE

Rapid changes in the attitudes of the purchasers of health services are producing responses from the provider community as well. The American health system is quickly moving away from delivery of health care through independent practitioners toward more integrated approaches. Perhaps the most important structural change now under way is the formation of integrated service delivery networks, such as physician-hospital organizations. Such networks market a comprehensive set of health services to health benefits plans, insurers and purchasers, and even directly to employers. They try to achieve savings through economies of scale and the coordination of patient care.

Much of the reorganization of health care is being prompted by the actions of insurers and managed care organizations, who themselves are competing for the health business of employers and other purchasers of care. Such organizations pursue the actual ownership or control of facilities and other capital resources and employ exclusive contracting with individual or groups of providers. Where they can, insurers and managed care organizations are capitalizing on the excess capacity in the health system (e.g., too many hospitals with too few patients) to negotiate favorable financial arrangements in exchange for serving groups of plan enrollees.

In other instances, providers are developing integrated systems independently by strengthening their own attractiveness in the marketplace. The scope of these efforts range from developing small groups of specialty providers into single organizations to comprehensive hospital and health systems that are prepared to compete to provide any and all services demanded in the market. Such systems often consist of hospitals, physicians and other practitioners, ambulatory care providers, and postacute facilities with the objective of eliminating some of the insurance overhead.

IMPLICATIONS FOR THE PROFESSION

The health marketplace is likely to remain in a state of flux, consolidation, and change for some time as the market forces described earlier bring about a major realignment of the resources needed to meet the health needs of the American people. Such change is causing a full-scale reexamination of the ways in which health providers have historically viewed their roles and futures and causing consumers to enter into different kinds of arrangements to obtain health care.

Providers are being asked to accept more stringent quality and utilization management monitoring, to accept competitively priced services, and to exercise more control over resource use. Consumers (i.e., patients) are being asked—and, in some cases, required—to accept that freedom to choose their providers in an oversupplied marketplace can no longer be guaranteed if they are to be assured access to health care at an affordable price.

In tomorrow's marketplace, payers will view workforce specialization as only adding cost and not enhancing quality—unless the rationale for such specialization is substantiated by real and convincing evidence.

In the past, quality assessment has often been based on the assumption that each procedure or service was necessary. This assumed that quality could be determined through evaluating structure, process, and outcome. However, many purchasers have begun to collect their own data that reveal enormous and unexplained variation in the practice styles of individual practitioners.

These buyers have also discovered that the professional literature often provides little, if any, information about the relative effectiveness, appropriateness, and costs of treatment alternatives. They have found, even where such information has been developed, that the recommendations contained in the literature or learned through experience in the classroom or clinic are not always reflected in the behavior of practitioners or in their practice styles.

Payers are likely to be especially skeptical about the provider-claimed benefits of certification and advanced training programs. Payers (and their purchasing agents) will focus on trying to get care delivered by the least trained people qualified to complete most of the tasks. They will attempt to employ, or contract with, a mix of trained individuals to provide the care, and not engage only the most educated or even the most experienced.

Many payers are relying increasingly on private accreditation programs (such as managed care plan accreditation offered by the National Committee for Quality Assurance) for addressing patient protection issues and the quality assurance aspects of care. Standards have been developed that address quality assurance, provider credentialing, utilization management, enrollee rights, and responsibilities.

> Health professionals must recognize that purchasers will be taking a much more aggressive role in designing the health plans of tomorrow.

With respect to the latter, plans meeting the standards must have policies recognizing such rights as voicing grievances and receiving information about the plan, its services, and its providers. Quality-related concerns are seen as going well beyond issues relating only to provider licensure and/or certification. They include systems for resolving member complaints and for collecting data for quality improvement purposes, including satisfaction surveys, provider "report cards," studies of reasons for disenrollment, and other policies and mechanisms for holding health plans and providers accountable to patients and purchasers.

Health professionals must recognize that purchasers will be taking a much more aggressive role in designing the health plans of tomorrow, and intend to use "smart" purchasing techniques that they employ in virtually all other aspects of their business. They start with the belief of American consumers and business that high quality and low cost are not inconsistent. More is not always better, but it is almost always more costly. ▼

8

A Brief History of Managed Care

The dominant focus of health care in the United States has been to provide service to the largest number of people. However, the focus has changed recently from *providing access* to *containing health care costs.*

Historically, the patient chose the physician, accepted whatever treatment was offered, and paid whatever fee was charged. Usually that wasn't a problem because if the patient had health insurance, the fees were either partially or fully covered under the insurance policy, which was often paid for by the patient's employer.

That payment system is called *fee for service.* Under this arrangement for health care delivery, patients, insurance companies, and employers had little to say about the fee charged or about the appropriateness or quality of the care.

However, the nation's health care system is rapidly changing from fee for service to *managed care.* What *is* managed care?

According to one definition, "managed care is a term used to describe health care systems that integrate the financing and delivery of appropriate health care services to covered individuals by arrangements with selected providers to furnish a comprehensive set of health care services, explicit standards for selection of health care providers, formal programs for ongoing quality assurance and utilization review, and significant financial incentives for members to use providers and procedures associated with the plan" (Harden, 1994).

Managed care is intended to address the issue of the skyrocketing cost of health care. According to the Congressional Budget Office, health care in 1992 cost the United States $838.5 billion, 14 percent of the nation's gross domestic product. By the year 2000, the nation's annual health care cost is expected to reach nearly $1.7 trillion—that's *18 percent* of the gross domestic product (Harden, 1994).

As a result of these costs, workers find themselves either paying higher percentages of their health insurance premiums or without any health insurance at all. As insurers, businesses, and consumers have become more concerned with the cost and availability of health care, they have begun demanding that care be accessible, appropriate, cost-effective, and of high quality. This has led to the widespread use of managed care.

The origins of managed care go back to 1929, when a physician in Elk City, Oklahoma (a town with only 6,000 residents and no medical specialists), established a rural farmers' cooperative health plan. The doctor sold shares of $50 each to raise money for a new hospital; he then provided each shareholder with medical care at a discounted rate. The annual dues schedule covered the cost of medical care, surgery, and house calls, as well as dental services. By 1934, the 600 family members of the cooperative supported the doctor, plus four specialists and a dentist.

Also in 1934, two physicians in Los Angeles entered into a prepaid contract to provide comprehensive health services to about 2,000 water company employees. These two plans were the beginning of the system known today as managed care.

From 1930 to 1960, several other prepaid group practice plans started up. Among them were: Group Health Association in Washington, D.C. (1937); the Kaiser-Permanente Medical Care Program (1942), the largest and best known health maintenance organization (HMO); the Group Health Cooperative of Puget Sound in Seattle (1947); the Health Insurance Plan of Greater New York (1947); and the Group Health Plan of Minneapolis (1957).

In 1954, a prototype individual practice association (IPA) was established by the San Joaquin County Foundation for Medical Care in Stockton, California. IPA/HMOs have grown more rapidly than either the group practice (a type of HMO where a single large multispecialty group practice is the sole—or major—source of care for an HMO's enrollees) or the staff model (where the majority of enrollees are cared for by physicians who are on the staff of the HMO) over the past 10–15 years.

It wasn't until 1972, however, that the term *HMO* was coined by Paul Ellwood for the Nixon administration. By 1973, only about five million people were enrolled in prepaid group practice plans. It is estimated that about 100 million people are now enrolled in managed care plans.

"The evolution of these pioneer prepaid group and individual practice plans in the private sector was one of the most extraordinary developments in the history of medical care organization in the world," says Gordon K. MacLeod, MD, FACP, Professor of Health Services Administration and Clinical Professor of Medicine at the University of Pittsburgh (1995).

"Prepaid plans went on to serve as a template for financing and organizing health care services for the American people; at the very least they ushered in a new era of corporate influence into the practice of medicine" (MacLeod, 1995).

Whether that is ultimately good or bad for the health care consumer, the provider, and the payer remains to be seen. However, on one point, everyone agrees: some form of managed care is probably here to stay. ▼

REFERENCES

Harden, S. L. (1994). *What legislators need to know about managed care.* Washington, DC: National Conference of State Legislatures.

MacLeod, G. K. (1995). An overview of managed health care. In P. R. Kongstvedt (Ed.), *Essentials of managed health care.* Gaithersburg, MD: Aspen Publishers.

A Glossary of Managed Care and Health Insurance Terms

This "Glossary of Managed Care and Health Insurance Terms" from the *Journal of Health Policy, Politics, and Law* is intended to provide occupational therapy practitioners with managed care and health insurance terminology that is commonly used across all sectors of the health care industry, including rehabilitation. It is not presented here as a comprehensive source of managed care terminology, but rather as a supplement to terms found in other areas of this resource guide.

As this glossary indicates, different terms are frequently used interchangeably to describe a similar managed care concept. The terms in this glossary, therefore, will not always completely match terms used in other articles contained in this resource guide.

Reprinted with permission from Duke University Press, "Raising a Tower of Babel— A Taxonomy of Managed Care and Health Insurance Plans" by Weiner and de Lissovy from *Journal of Health Politics, Policy, and Law*, Vol. 18, No. 1, Spring 1993.

▼   ▼   ▼

Alternative delivery system (ADS): A generic term for new systems seen as alternatives to traditional fee-for-service indemnity health insurance plans. ADSs usually involve a significant degree of integration between payer and providers. The ADS entity is legally committed to provide care or to arrange for its provision through a network of providers. The ADS entity also manages this care. The two major types of ADSs are HMOs and PPOs. ADSs are rapidly becoming mainstream; the term *alternative* is somewhat of a misnomer and is being used less frequently. We propose the term *integrated delivery system*. (See also *HMO, managed care, PPO*.)

Carve-out plan: See *single-benefit plan*.

Case management (CM): (1) An arrangement in which a "case manager" who is not a physician (usually a registered nurse or master of social work) serves as a medical ombudsman responsible for coordinating the care process for selected consumers. Case managers usually work with patients having expensive conditions (e.g., those with AIDS or cancer, and premature neonates). We suggest that this is the appropriate use of the term. (2) Sometimes used interchangeably with *managed care.* (3) An arrangement where a "gatekeeper" physician must deliver or approve the delivery of all care. (See *coordinated care* and *gatekeeper.*)

Competitive medical plan (CMP): A term used by the U.S. Health Care Financing Administration (HCFA) for a subset of the organizations that have "risk contracts" to serve Medicare beneficiaries on a capitated payment basis (based on an adjusted average per capita cost, or AAPCC). HCFA does not consider these organizations to be HMOs because they are not federally qualified (by HCFA's Office of Prepaid Health Care, OPHC). This term is sometimes used interchangeably with ADS.

Coordinated care: A term HCFA often uses more or less generically for managed care plans, particularly if they use gatekeepers.

Exclusive provider organization (EPO): A type of PPO in which the patient must "exclusively" use the providers within the PPO. This characteristic is sometimes called a *lock-in provision.* If the EPO entity bears risk that is directly related to utilization of its enrollees, it can be categorized as a *risk-sharing EPO* or *R/EPO.* (See *PPO* and *R/EPO.*)

Gatekeeper: A primary care physician (i.e., a family practitioner, internist, or pediatrician) who is responsible for coordinating *all* services. In a gatekeeper plan, most elective specialist or hospital care cannot be delivered without the gatekeeper's approval. This system is used by most HMOs and EPOs. In HMOs, the gatekeeper is usually placed at financial risk for referral and hospital care, a condition that serves as a disincentive to "open the gate." In non-HMOs, the gatekeeper does not share risk and is paid separately for gatekeeper services. State Medicaid programs use this approach fairly extensively and often label gatekeeper physicians *case managers.* There have been some instances of physicians forming networks to offer their coordinating services to integrated delivery systems that choose to purchase them. Such freestanding groups of gatekeepers have sometimes been called *primary care networks.* (See also *case management.*)

Group-model HMO: A type of HMO in which a single large multispecialty group practice is the sole (or major) source of care for an HMO's enrollees. The group may or may not have existed before the corporately distinct HMO entity formed, but it has an exclusive contract only with the one HMO. Some groups also see fee-for-service or PPO patients; others are not allowed to do so. Because of the similarity with the staff-model HMO, the term *staff/group-model HMO* is often used to denote these large HMOs. (See also *HMO* and *network-model HMO.*)

Health-insuring organization (HIO): See *risk-sharing EPO.*

Health maintenance organization (HMO): A prepaid organized delivery system in which the organization and the primary care physicians assume some financial risk for the care provided to its enrolled members. Often, the physicians serving HMO patients are paid on a capitation basis. The HMO is legally committed to provide care to its enrollees. In a *pure* HMO, members must obtain care from within the system if it is to be reimbursed.

The term *HMO* was coined by Paul Ellwood for the Nixon administration in 1972. This constituted a renaming of two existing delivery models: prepaid group practices (PPGPs), or closed-panel plans, and independent practice associations (IPAs), or open-panel plans. (The panel refers to the panel of physicians available to the member.) The earliest PPGPs were often founded by socially conscious consumer collectives patterned loosely after European sick funds. In most of the early HMOs, the financing and delivery of care were very closely integrated. For example, these HMOs did not reimburse physicians for their services, they hired them directly. Today, there are four basic HMO models (staff, group, network, and IPA) and several related variants and hybrids. (See also *group-model HMO, IPA, mixed-model HMO, network-model HMO, O/HMO, risk-sharing EPO, S/HMO,* and *staff-model HMO.*)

Hybrid health plan: See *point-of-service plan.*

Independent practice association or **individual practice association (IPA):** An open-panel type of HMO in which individual physicians (or small group practices) contract to provide care to enrolled members. The primary care physicians may be paid by capitation, or by fee for service with a "with-hold" risk-sharing provision. An IPA entity may or may not be legally distinct from the HMO entity with which the member enrolls. Physicians participating in IPAs retain their right to treat non-HMO patients on a fee-for-service basis. Most of the early IPAs were developed by organized medicine to compete with large closed-panel HMOs. Many of these initial plans were sponsored by local medical societies and were known as *foundations for medical care (FMCs).* (Many FMCs also were the sites of early *professional standards review organizations, PSROs.* See also *HMO* and *network-model HMO.*)

Integrated delivery system: See *alternative delivery system.*

Managed care: A term often used generically for all types of integrated delivery systems, such as HMOs and PPOs, implying that they "manage" the care received by consumers (in contrast to traditional fee-for-service care, which is "unmanaged"). More recently, this term is used to denote the entire range of utilization control tools that are applied to manage the practices of physicians and others, regardless of the setting in which they practice.

In addition to being used in all HMOs, PPOs, and EPOs, these controls are increasingly being applied to conventional fee-for-service indemnity plans (see *managed indemnity plan*). The types of methods used to manage the patient's care may include preadmission certification, mandatory second opinion before surgery, certification of treatment plans for discretionary nonemergency services (such as mental health care), primary care physician gatekeepers and nonphysician case managers to monitor the care of particular patients. The actual managing organization is frequently an entity separate from the payer or insurer.

Among managed indemnity plans, this type of organization is often called a *managed care company*, or *third-party administrator* (see *TPA*). The term *managed care* is sometimes used (especially among Medicaid agencies) to denote a case manager program. (Also see *ADS, case management, coordinated care, MIP*.)

Managed competition: A model proposed for national health care reform in which independent plans (primarily, integrated managed care plans) compete with one another in a market closely regulated by government. In this case, it is the health plan that is being "managed."

Managed indemnity plan (MIP): A type of health plan in which the insurer (or its agent) uses a significant number of utilization controls to manage the practices of providers it reimburses. These controls are more extensive than those used in traditional indemnity plans. Providers are paid on a fee-for-service basis and a variety of mechanisms may be used to determine rates of payment. A plan is not usually considered an MIP if it does not mandate preadmission certification for elective hospitalizations. (See also *managed care*.)

16

Medicare-insured group (MIG): See *R/EPO*.

MeSH (medical staff and hospital): A joint venture, in which a hospital (or hospitals) and its private practice medical staff (or other body of independent physicians) form a corporation. The MeSH entity, as a unit, may then contract to provide in-patient and/or ambulatory care to patients enrolled in an HMO or PPO (which is corporately distinct from the MeSH). The MeSH can also become a PPO or HMO by negotiating directly with employer groups or payers and by relating to outside providers on a contractual basis.

Mixed-model HMO: An HMO that is a mixture of the relatively distinct staff, group, network, or independent practice association (IPA) varieties. For example, an HMO that serves a significant proportion of its enrollees within a staff model site but also contracts with several other groups or IPA entities may be of this type. An HMO can be a mixed model when assessed within a particular market area or across areas. These types of HMOs are becoming more common, as HMOs of one model acquire or merge with previously distinct HMOs of a different type. The results of such mergers are frequently known as *network-model HMOs*. (See also *network-model HMO* and *O/HMO*.)

Network-model HMO: A type of HMO in which a network of two or more existing group practices has contracted to care for the majority of patients enrolled in an HMO plan. A network-model HMO also sometimes contracts with individual providers in a fashion similar to an IPA. Providers contracting with this type of HMO are usually free to serve fee-for-service patients as well as those enrolled in other HMOs and PPOs. The term *network/IPA* is often used to encompass both this and the IPA HMOs. (See also *HMO* and *IPA*.)

Open-ended HMO or **open HMO (O/HMO):** A type of HMO in which the enrollees are not "locked in"; they may leave the HMO and still have certain services covered. Such "out-of-plan" use is usually subject to a significant degree of cost sharing (e.g., deductibles), unlike those services delivered within the plan. The out-of-plan segment of HMO use may fall within an existing nonmanaged indemnity plan, MIP, or PPO run by the HMO or its parent corporation.

To be considered an O/HMO, the plan must retain all risk and the primary care physicians must share in that risk. This usually includes the risk associated with out-of-plan use. These plans are sometime termed *point-of-service (POS) HMOs, hybrid HMOs, HMO swing-outs,* and *flexible HMOs.* (Plans using these labels often share some risk with employers.) Currently, this class of plan is still somewhat loosely defined. Many point-of-service plans, which are not linked to an existing pure HMO, would more accurately be classified as PPOs or a type of triple-option plan (TOP). (See also *PPO* and *TOP.*)

Point-of-service (POS) plan: A hybridized managed care plan that offers the consumer a choice of options at the time he or she seeks services (rather than at the time he or she chooses to enroll in a health plan). There are (at least) three types of POS plans: (1) an open-ended HMO, (2) a triple-option plan, and (3) a "unified" PPO. POS plans are also known as *flexible health plans, mixed-model health plans,* or *hybrid model plans.* (See *O/HMO, PPO,* and *TOP.*)

Preferred provider arrangement (PPA): Similar to a PPO, except purchasers selectively contract directly with a provider, usually without benefit of a comprehensive administrative entity like a PPO. Usually, no significant managing of care takes place in PPAs. (See also *PPO.*)

Preferred provider organization (PPO): A type of integrated delivery system in which the PPO entity acts as a broker between the purchaser of care and the provider. In a PPO, consumers have the option of using the "preferred" providers available within the plan, or not. Consumers are channeled toward in-plan providers by incentives and disincentives (relating to cost-sharing provisions and benefit coverage). In return for the patient referrals, providers agree that their care will be "managed." Providers usually received a discounted fee-for-service payment (e.g., 80 percent of their usual fee) and they do not participate in financial risk sharing. A "unified" PPO is a plan that bears risk for both in-plan and out-of-plan use. These plans are sometimes marketed as point-of-service plans. (See also *EPO* and *POS plan.*)

Risk-sharing exclusive provider organization (R/EPO): An exclusive provider organization (see *EPO*) in which the organization shares a significant amount of risk with the payer.
Unlike an IPA-type HMO, the R/EPO does *not* share any of this risk with its primary care
physicians (e.g., via capitation or withholds). A health insurance organization (HIO) was a
type of R/EPO. It was a plan developed to contract with a state's Medicaid administration to
provide care on a prepaid basis only to Medicaid enrollees. Legislation all but eliminated
these and other plans serving 100 percent Medicaid enrollees. Another prototype plan
proposed for Medicare beneficiaries and known as *Medicare-insured groups (MIGs)*, is also a
type of R/EPO. MIGs are collectives of Medicare beneficiaries, such as union- or employer-
related groups, that receive a predetermined capitation amount for a defined population of
beneficiaries. The MIG assumes all risk for purchasing the care for those enrolled.

Single-benefit plan: An entity that subcontracts with other organizations—for example,
HMOs, indemnity insurers, or EPOs (usually on a capitated basis)—to provide health
services only within a "single benefit" category. Single benefit plans have been set up to
provide mental health, dental, or eye care only. The providers in these plans may or may not
participate in risk-sharing arrangements, but the plan itself is usually at full risk for the services it contracts to provide. These plans are often termed *carve-out plans*, because selected
services are carved out of the full array of coverage offered by the main insurer. (Also known
as *single-benefit HMOs*.)

Social HMO (S/HMO): A type of HMO developed mainly on a demonstration basis with
HCFA funding. It is intended to expand traditional HMO medical services to provide social
support and long-term care to the elderly and disabled enrollees. The S/HMO arrangement
may revolve around a conventional HMO that contracts with a long-term care provider, a
long-term care agency that contracts with medical providers, or an independent broker that
contracts with all providers. (See also *HMO*.)

Staff-model HMO: A type of HMO in which the majority of enrollees is cared for by
physicians who are on the staff of the HMO. Although these physicians may be involved in
risk-sharing arrangements, a majority of their income is usually derived from a fixed salary.
The "group cooperative" consumer-controlled HMOs are usually staff-model plans. Because
the physicians in this type of HMO are also organized in groups, the label *group/staff-model*
is used to encompass both this and the group-model HMO. (See also *group-model HMO*
and *HMO*.)

Third-party administrator (TPA): A private firm that serves as the agent or intermediary
of a health plan when dealing with providers. These firms can be considered distinct corporate entities, separate from the health plan or insurer. (Through sister or parent corpora-
tions, however, many TPAs do offer their own health plans.) TPAs are responsible for at

least some (if not all) administrative functions, but a TPA bears no financial risk associated with the insurance function. Some TPAs handle the claims payment process. Many TPAs manage the care paid for by the at-risk entity (e.g., the plan or employer). A TPA performing this function is often known as a *managed care* or *utilization review (UR) company.* TPAs are most frequently retained by self-insured employers, but increasingly, nationally oriented managed indemnity plans, PPOs, independent practice associations, and point-of-service plans are using their services. (See also *managed care.*)

Triple-option plan (TOP): A "single" plan (or a collection of contractually linked freestanding plans) that offers a consumer the choice of three health benefit options at the time of enrollment. TOPs offer an HMO, a PPO, and a managed indemnity plan (or a nonmanaged indemnity plan) under the same corporate umbrella. TOPs are often coordinated or owned by insurers who have formed or acquired freestanding HMOs or PPOs. To be considered a TOP, the risk for all plan options must be retained by a single entity. To an employer, a key advantage of a TOP (vs. nonlinked plans offered to employees by separate insurers) is that the issue of "biased selection," where healthier employees select one plan over another, is avoided; the same insurer bears the risk, regardless of which plan an employee chooses. A TOP that offers the consumer three choices at the point of service (rather than at the time of enrollment) is usually termed a *point-of-service plan.* (See also *POS plan.*)

INSURANCE ACRONYMS AND DEFINITIONS

Accreditation: The process by which a government or nongovernment agency evaluates and recognizes an individual, institution, or educational program as meeting predetermined standards.

Actual charge: The health care provider's billed or submitted charge.

Allowable charge: The maximum fee that a third party will use to reimburse a provider for a given service.

Assignment (Medicare): Term for the Medicare-approved amount (including the 80 percent Medicare payment and 20 percent patient co-payment) paid to a health care provider.

Balance bill: That portion of a health care provider's charge exceeding the Medicare-approved amount, which is billed to the patient. The patient is responsible for the 20 percent co-payment and the amount of the health care provider's charge that exceeds the Medicare-approved amount up to the limiting charge. Only nonparticipating health care providers may balance bill their Medicare patients.

Benefit: A sum of money that an insurance policy pays for covered services, under the terms of the policy.

Benefit period: The time during which an insurance policy provides payments for covered benefits.

Blue Cross/Blue Shield Association (BC/BS): A nationwide federation of local, nonprofit insurance organizations that contract with hospitals and other health care providers to make payments for health care services to their subscribers.

Budget neutrality: A provision of the Omnibus Budget Reconciliation Act of 1989, the legislation creating the Medicare RBRVS payment system, that requires that expenditures resulting from changes in medical practice or payment methodology neither increase nor decrease from what they would have been under a continuation of the customary, prevailing, and reasonable charge system.

Capitation: A method of payment for health services in which a provider receives a fixed, prepaid, per capita amount for each person enrolled in the health plan for whom the provider has responsibility for all necessary health care services.

Carrier (Medicare): A private contractor to HCFA that administers claims processing and payment for Medicare Part B services.

Case management: A component of many insurance programs designed to ensure that appropriate and necessary medical and rehabilitation services are provided to specific patients in a cost-effective manner. A case manager generally coordinates all services required by a particular patient and acts as both an advocate for the patient and an agent of the payer.

Catastrophic health insurance: A type of health insurance that provides protection against the high cost of treating severe or lengthy illnesses or disabilities.

CHAMPUS: Civilian Health and Medical Program of the Uniformed Services. A program paid for by the Department of Defense that pays for care that civilian health providers deliver to retired members and dependents of active and retired military personnel. This program does not charge premiums but has cost-sharing provisions.

Claim: A request to an insurer for payment of benefits under an insurance policy.

Claim adjudication: The determination of payment on a claim based on type of contract, type of coverage, and present use.

Coinsurance: The component of a health insurance plan that requires the insurer and patient each to pay a percentage of covered costs. For example, in an 80 percent/20 percent plan, the insurer pays 80 percent of the allowable charge (after the patient has paid the deductible) and the insured person pays 20 percent.

Consumer price index (CPI): Published by the U.S. Department of Labor, a measure of increases in the price of a market basket of goods and services by region of the country.

Contributory insurance: Type of group insurance in which the employee pays for all or part of the premium and the employer or union pays the remainder.

Coordination of benefits (COB): Provisions and procedures that insurers use to avoid duplicative payments for claims when a person has more than one insurance policy.

Co-payment: A specified amount of money per visit or unit of time that the patient pays, while the insurer pays the rest of the claim.

Cost sharing: The requirement in health insurance plans for the patient to pay part of the cost of care. Cost-sharing arrangements include deductibles, coinsurance, user fees, and shared premiums.

CPT: [Physicians'] Current Procedural Terminology coding manual published by the American Medical Association.

Deductible: The amount of loss or expense that an insured or covered individual must incur before an insurer assumes any liability for all or part of the remaining cost of covered services.

Department of Health and Human Services (HHS): Department within the U.S. government that is responsible for administering health and social welfare programs.

Dependent: A person who can be claimed on insurance. Dependents can include a policy-holder's spouse and unmarried children who meet eligibility requirements.

Diagnosis-related groups (DRGs): Classifications of illnesses and injuries that are used as the basis for prospective payments to hospitals under Medicare and other insurers.

Durable medical equipment, prosthetics, orthotics, and supplies (DMEPOS): Medically necessary equipment and supplies, such as oxygen equipment, wheelchairs, braces, or splints, that a health care provider prescribes for a patient's home use.

Fee-for-service: A payment method by which a health care provider is reimbursed for each encounter or service rendered.

Fee schedule: A list of accepted charges or established allowances for specified medical or dental procedures.

Group insurance: An insurance plan in which a number of employees and their dependents are insured under a single policy.

HCFA: Health Care Financing Administration. The agency under the Department of Health and Human Services that is responsible for administering major health care programs, including the Medicare and Medicaid programs.

HCPCS: HCFA Common Procedure Coding System. Level 1 (CPT) and level 2 (alphanumeric HCPCS).

Health care provider: Any person, firm, corporation, partnership, association, agency, institution, or other legal entity providing any kind of health care–related services. "Providers" include, but are not limited to, physicians, dentists, chiropractors, vocational rehabilitation counselors, osteopaths, pharmacists, physicians, podiatrists, occupational therapists, physical therapists, psychologists, durable medical equipment dealers, psychiatric social workers, optometrists, registered nurses, licensed practical nurses, acupuncturists, Christian Science practitioners, and institutions such as hospitals, clinics, rehabilitation facilities, home health agencies, nursing facilities, and outpatient surgery centers.

Health professional shortage areas (HPSAs): Urban or rural areas identified by the Public Health Service (PHS) as being medically underserved. The PHS may also designate population groups and public nonprofit private medical facilities as medically underserved. Physicians in designated HPSAs who furnish covered services to Medicare patients receive a 10 percent bonus payment in addition to the payment schedule amount.

HMO: Health maintenance organization. A type of insurance program that provides health care in a geographic area with a standardized set of basic and supplemental health services. This type of program serves a group, with each member prepaying a fixed amount per year to receive all required medical care.

Insured: The individual or organization protected in the case of loss under the terms of an insurance policy.

Insurer: The party that contracts to pay losses or render services for an insurance policy.

IPA: Independent practice association. A partnership, corporation, association, or other legal entity that has entered into an arrangement for provision of its services with persons who are licensed to practice medicine.

Limiting charge: Statutory limit on the amount a nonparticipating health care provider can charge for services to Medicare patients. The limiting charge for 1993 and all subsequent years is 115 percent of the Medicare-approved amount for nonparticipating providers.

Locality: Geographic areas defined by HCFA and used to establish payment amounts for physician services. There are currently 217 Medicare localities nationwide. Some localities are states; others are counties or groups of counties.

Major medical insurance: A type of insurance designed to offset the heavy medical expenses resulting from a prolonged illness or injury.

Managed care: A health care cost containment approach that enables the payer to influence the delivery of health services prospectively (i.e., before services are provided). Techniques used by managed care programs include case management, physician gatekeepers, provider networks, and components of utilization review, such as admission review, discharge planning, and mandatory second-opinion programs.

Medicaid: A health insurance program administered jointly by state and federal governments for low-income persons, regardless of age.

Medical fee schedule: A list that establishes the recommended maximum level of reimbursement for medical services. Some fee schedules list actual dollar amounts, while others are based on formulas and may include limitations on the number of units of service, restrictions on the frequency of service, requirements for the treatment plans, or requirements for referrals.

Medicare: A nationwide health insurance program administered by HCFA for persons aged 65 and over, disabled, or those with chronic kidney disease.

Medicare payment schedule (also see RBRVS): A payment schedule adopted by HCFA for payment of physician and independent practitioner services effective January 1, 1992, replacing the customary, prevailing, and reasonable system. This payment schedule is based on the resource costs of health care provider work, practice overhead, and professional liability insurance, with adjustments for differences in geographic practice costs. The payment schedule amount for a service includes both the 80 percent that Medicare pays and the patient's 20 percent co-payment.

Medigap policy: A type of insurance that is sold by private insurance companies that covers medical expenses not covered by Medicare.

Nonparticipating health care provider: A health care provider who has not signed a participation agreement with Medicare and is, therefore, not obligated to accept the Medicare-approved amount as payment in full for all cases. Nonparticipating providers may still accept assignment on a case-by-case basis. Nonparticipating providers bill Medicare patients directly, including the balance of the charge that is not covered by the Medicare-approved amount. However, this balance cannot exceed the limiting charge.

Open enrollment period: A period of time in which new subscribers may elect to enroll in a health insurance plan. During this time, previously enrolled subscribers may switch from one health plan to another without any penalties.

Out-of-pocket payment or costs: Costs borne solely by a patient without benefit of insurance.

Palliative care: Care rendered to *temporarily* reduce or moderate the intensity of an otherwise chronic medical condition.

Participating health care provider (Medicare): A health care provider who has signed a participation agreement with Medicare. A participating provider is bound by the agreement to accept assignment on all Medicare claims for a calendar year.

Per diem rate: A fixed all-inclusive price for one day of hospital or nursing facility care, including all supplies and services provided to the patient during a day, excluding the professional fees of nonstaff physicians.

Physician Payment Review Commission (PPRC): An advisory body created by Congress in 1986 to recommend reforms in the methods Medicare used to pay for physician and nonphysician practitioner services.

Physician/therapist work (Medicare): Under the resource-based relative value scale (RBRVS) payment system instructions, the physician's/therapist's individual effort in providing a service, including time, technical difficulty of the procedure, severity of patient's condition, and the physical and mental effort required to provide the service; one of three resource cost components included in the formula for computing Medicare payment schedule amounts.

PPO: Preferred provider organization. A network of medical care providers and facilities that agree to discount their charges in return for a high volume of patients. Employers may agree to channel their employees to a PPO network to receive a lower insurance premium. Employees can use providers outside the PPO but are encouraged not to do so by lower out-of-pocket costs for deductibles and coinsurances.

Practice expense (Medicare): Under RBRVS instructions, the cost of health care provider practice overhead, including rent, staff salaries and benefits, medical equipment, and supplies; one of three resource cost components included in the formula for computing Medicare
payment schedule amounts.

Premium: The amount paid to an insurer or third party for insurance coverage under an insurance policy.

Preventive medicine: Care designed to deter disease and maintain optimal health.

Primary care provider: A clinician who assumes ongoing responsibility for a patient's overall health care needs.

Professional liability (malpractice) insurance: Insurance to protect a health care provider against professional liability. Under RBRVS instructions, one of three resource cost components included in the formula developed by HCFA for computing Medicare payment schedule amounts.

Provider: The person or organization, such as the physician, therapist, hospital, or health maintenance organization, who actually provides the health care.

RBRVS: Resource-based relative value scale. Medicare's system for payment to physicians and independent practitioners where the relative values for practitioner work, practice, and malpractice are multiplied by a specific conversion factor to compute a payment amount.

RUC: RVS Update Committee. An American Medical Association committee that recommends relative value weights to HCFA for the Medicare RBRVS fee schedule.

RVS: Relative value scale. An index of practitioner's services ranked according to the "value" of the service. In a charge-based RVS, services are ranked according to the average fee for the service. A resource-based RVS ranks services according to the relative value costs of the resources required.

RVU: Relative value unit. The unit of measure for Medicare resource-based relative value scale. RVUs must be multiplied by a dollar conversion factor to determine payment amounts.

25

Self-insure: The practice of an individual, group, employer, or organization assuming complete responsibility for losses that might be incurred, such as medical costs, rather than purchasing insurance.

Supplemental health insurance: A type of health insurance that reimburses the policyholder for services that are not reimbursed by the policyholder's primary health insurance. (See *Medigap policy*.)

Third-party payer: A group that pays or insures health or medical expenses on behalf of beneficiaries.

Underwrite: The practice of an insurer assuming the financial risk of an insurance policy for a person or group of people.

Usual, customary, and reasonable (UCR): The average charge for a similar medical service by providers in a specific geographical area.

Utilization review: A series of individual reviews conducted to ensure that a patient is not unnecessarily admitted to a hospital nor receives inappropriate care.

Workers' compensation law: A law that requires employers to furnish benefits and health care to employees injured on the job and to pay benefits to dependents of employees who are killed on the job. Workers' Compensation is mandatory in most states.

Critical Pathways

INTRODUCTION

"A critical path is an optimal, sequencing and timing of interventions by physicians, nurses, and other staff for a particular diagnosis or procedure, designed to minimize the delays and resource utilization and to maximize the quality of care" (Coffey et al., 1992). The critical path methodology, or CPM, has its origins in the fields of construction and engineering. As a management tool within these industries, it has been used to track completion times and other data related to large, complex projects.

Although some of the concepts related to critical paths were discussed within the health care industry in the 1970s, it was not until the 1980s that the health care environment was receptive to incorporating such an approach into clinical practice. Environmental factors influencing this change included

- ▼ the introduction of a prospective payment system for reimbursing acute inpatient hospitalization;

- ▼ increasing evidence of wide variation in the delivery of care and related outcomes;

- ▼ increasing malpractice costs and an emphasis on defensive medicine; and

- ▼ increasing involvement by a number of providers and professionals in the delivery of care to individual patients.

In other parts of industrial America, the quality control movement was receiving increased attention. Emphasis was being placed on the need for organizations to focus on reducing variations in how things were done and to look at improvement from a systems perspective to produce quality outcomes.

As stated above, with the advent of diagnosis-related groups and accreditation standards that focused on quality improvement, hospitals became cognizant of the need to find mechanisms to maximize efficiency and effectiveness in the delivery of services. Similarly, in our current climate finding methods of delivering high-quality patient care while controlling costs may be the ultimate challenge facing health care providers in the 1990s.

Like many new processes in quality improvement, clinical paths took time to catch on. Reservations about the use of clinical paths were expressed by physicians and other health care providers, who perceived the use of clinical paths as cookbook practice, questioned legal ramifications of their use, and resented the work required to develop them. However, an increasing number of hospitals, health care organizations, and providers are realizing that clinical pathways are one of the essential foundations of a total quality management process as well as a tool for case management activities and to help "manage care" within certain case types.

Critical work on adapting the CPM into the acute care setting took place in 1985 at the New England Medical Center (Zander, 1993). Today, this tool is an integral part of patient care management with various populations and within a wide range of settings where occupational therapy services are provided. In addition, organizations such as the Center for Case Management provide valuable resources to the beginner as well as the seasoned professional.

DEFINITIONS

Various terms are used to describe methods to achieve coordinated care. Often called clinical pathways, care maps, care plans, or critical pathways, several noted experts have provided definitions for these terms:

▼ Patrice Spath defines critical paths as "a description of key events in the process of care which should be accomplished to achieve maximum quality at minimal costs" (Spath, 1993).

▼ As stated previously, Richard Coffey et al. (1992) define critical paths as "an optimal sequencing and timing of interventions by physicians, nurses, and other staff for a particular diagnosis or procedure."

▼ Karen Zander defines her CareMap tools (CareMaps™)[1] as "a cause-and-effect grid which identifies expected patient/family and staff behaviors against a time line for a case type or otherwise defined homogenous population" (Zander, 1992). Components of a CareMap include a time line, an index of problems with intermediate goals and outcome criteria, a critical path, and a variance record.

---

[1]The term CareMap™ is a registered trademark, and only those organizations trained by the Center for Case Management are licensed to use the term.

▼ Robin Underwood in her AOTA on-line workshop (AOTA, 1995) sees merit in all these definitions and feels that how the specific tool is defined and developed depends upon the needs of the individual organization. She states that the most relevant point is that "critical pathways are an indication of the course of patient treatment on a time line, with an outcome orientation, and with prompts for a multidisciplinary staff to perform important interventions so that costs are contained and quality, as defined by the consumers, is assured…. It is a layout or road map of what is to be accomplished within defined times by each member of the clinical team during a predetermined estimated length of stay or number of treatments."

DEVELOPING CRITICAL PATHWAYS

The process for development and use of critical paths will vary among organizations. However, the following steps are typically involved:

(1) Selecting a diagnosis or procedure for development—Selection can be based on factors such as volume, financial impact, payer, or referral interest. Different pathways within certain diagnoses may need to be developed separately due to factors such as age, clinical variability, or treatment protocols.

(2) Determining development team composition—Successful team composition is a major consideration. Consistent with other quality improvement projects, the team should include all disciplines involved in the selected diagnosis or procedure. In addition, consideration needs to be given to representation from the different professional levels as well as from different settings along the continuum. As pathways become an integral part of documentation and, in some cases, computerized records, it is essential in these situations to involve representatives from information systems.

(3) Defining current practice—The team needs to define and document current practice, procedures, medications, teaching, and the timing of aspects of care, along with outcomes. This can be done through chart review and team meetings.

(4) Researching internal and external practices—This involves the investigation of practice variations and, as available, review of pathways from other organizations. Critical questions need to be asked on the whys of current practice and how things could be done more efficiently and effectively.

(5) Writing the critical pathway—Based on the actions above, the multidisciplinary team writes the critical path. This includes defining measures, outcomes, process items, timeliness, and variations from the path.

(6) Implementing the critical path—In most instances, the team that develops the path should be the one to implement it. Many times an individual within an institution (e.g., an internal case manager) is designated to track adherence to the path, variances, and problems with achieving desired outcomes.

(7) Collecting the processing date—How data will be collected, who will collect the data, and how the data will be used need to be determined.

(8) Educating staff—Staff involved with implementing the critical pathway need to be oriented regarding its use, data collection, documentation, variances, and other features.

(9) Analyzing results—Critical pathways contain a gold mine of information. Results for analysis include length of stay, variations from the pathway, resource use, and outcomes.

(10) Improving the path and continuous monitoring—Based on analyses and changes in clinical practice, pathway modification should take place. This is a key benefit of using a tool consistent with quality management principles.

CONCEPTS AND COMPONENTS

Regardless of the term used, critical pathways have several distinct features, as described by Coffey et al. (1992):

(1) Comprehensiveness—Inherent in a pathway are the activities, services, and coordinated actions among all providers involved in the care of patients defined by the critical pathway.

(2) Time lines—Specified time lines are delineated for each intervention and patient care activity.

(3) Collaboration—Path development is accomplished by a multidisciplinary team of professionals.

(4) Patient management—Patients being managed on a critical pathway usually have a case coordinator or case manager to oversee the process.

FORMAT

The typical format for most critical pathways is a matrix of activities by day or hour (depending upon the setting and application). Several commercial models are available. However, it is important to customize "off-the-shelf" pathways or those of other institutions and organizations and to individualize them for one's own setting or practice for successful implementation and use.

CATEGORIES

In addition to specifying time frames, patient care activities and interventions are organized into categories. Examples may include consults, assessments, medications, nutrition, patient/family education, treatments, and discharge planning. These categories will vary depending upon the setting and environment. It is important to note that such categories and items describe the treatment process or specific tasks carried out by providers at specified time periods or intervals outlined on the path. In essence, the pathway becomes a visual display of the treatment process over the patient's length of stay.

OUTCOMES

In addition to process items or types of interventions, another important consideration is the inclusion of patient-related clinical outcomes within the clinical pathway. This allows all parties involved, including the patient and family, to track progress and outcomes along with the care provided. As the managed care industry focuses on the use of critical pathways, they can be a potentially valuable marketing tool. By including all these dimensions, one can demonstrate a focus on controlling length of stay, resource use, and patient outcomes. This is a well-balanced picture of both sides of the equation, that is, cost and quality.

31

VARIANCE

Because pathways are written for the "typical" patient or majority of patients falling within a designated category, variances or deviations from the critical pathway will occur. Deviations can be related to any of the components outlined above and can result in changes in length of stay, costs, and outcomes. Variances may be positive (e.g. a patient making more and quicker progress than specified on the pathway) or negative (e.g., activities cannot be completed or outcomes cannot be achieved within the pathway's time frames). Variances may be avoidable or unavoidable. They may be related to the patient, the clinician, or a system failure. Regardless of the underlying factor(s), variances must be documented. Tracking and analyzing variances and instituting corrective action are critical components of the entire process.

DOCUMENTATION

One of the major objectives for developing critical pathways is to streamline documentation. Critical pathways may or may not be included as part of a permanent medical record. Ideally, they should be to save time as well as avoid redundance and duplication with documentation and entering information into the medical record. Unless one's system is totally integrated and computerized, some duplicate documentation related to the critical paths is inevitable.

CONCLUSION

Critical paths are being developed and integrated into more institutions and used by health care providers. A summary of the benefits and uses include the following:

(1) an integrated, coordinated plan of care;

(2) increased multidisciplinary collaboration;

(3) reduced variation in the care process;

(4) education and orientation of staff, patients, and families;

(5) reduced lengths of stay, resource use, and related costs;

(6) enhanced communication internally and externally; and

(7) quality improvement and quality outcomes.

Critical pathways are a powerful tool in today's evolving health care environment. They are consistent with and complement the goal of being responsive to issues of cost containment, decreasing variations in the delivery of services, and ensuring and maintaining high quality outcomes.

Although many feel that managed care companies are focusing exclusively on cost as the primary factor in today's marketplace, it is up to all of us as providers and consumers of health care services to recognize and emphasize the importance of quality in this equation. ▼

REFERENCES

Coffey, R., Richards, J., Remmert, C., LeRoy, S., Schoville, R., & Baldwin, P. (1992). An introduction to critical paths. *Quality Management in Health Care 1* (1), 45–54.

Joe, B.E. (1996). Is there an OT role in acute care? *OT Week*, 10 (6), 12-13.

Spath, P. (Ed.). (1994). *Clinical tools for outcomes management.* Chicago: AHA Publications.

Zander, K. (1993a). *D.E.F.I.N.I.T.I.O.N., the first five years.* South Natick, MA: Center for Case Management.

Zander, K. (1993B). *The new definition: Prelude to restructuring.* South Natick, MA: Center for Case Management.

Report Cards

INTRODUCTION

The concept of assessing quality in health care is not new. Such activities have been performed by providers and organizations for years, primarily due to requirements from the government, accrediting agencies, and third-party payers. On occasion, an institution carried out these activities on its own initiative. However, other than knowing that an organization was licensed or accredited, results of quality-related programs were kept confidential and no method existed for determining which organization provided the "best health care."

In the mid-1980s, there was a push by corporate purchasers to evaluate health care quality and to get the most value for their money. Employers were battling rising health care costs, and it was essential to hold health plans accountable for their performance. The old responses "trust me" and "we're doing the best we can" just weren't enough justification anymore. Attempts were made to work with health care organizations, primarily managed care plans, to develop information sets to facilitate purchasing decisions. Difficulty arose over which performance indicators to use.

More recently, in concert with sentiments that publishing quality of care results could contain health care expenditures, several states (California, New York, Pennsylvania) and health care plans (Harvard Community Health Plan, Kaiser Permanente, U.S. Healthcare) have begun publishing reports on health care provided by their respective hospitals and plans. Published summaries of health plan (or hospital) performance indicators are being called report cards.

LIMITATIONS AND BENEFITS

Limitations—According to a U. S. General Accounting Office publication on the subject of report cards, it is felt that report cards can be useful to educate external audiences and stakeholders about the costs, care, and quality provided by competing health plans. This is viewed as a positive step toward containing costs and emphasizing quality outcomes. However, there are many obstacles to using report cards, as outlined in this report. These include "(1) inaccurate, misleading, or incomplete information sources; (2) indicators that may not measure quality; (3) little agreement on formulas for calculating performance results; and (4) no verification mechanisms in place to ensure the accuracy of reported results" (U. S. General Accounting Office, 1994).

For instance, the current indicators measure organizational structure or activities carried out by providers (i.e., process items). Typical items may include number of mammograms, immunization rates, or mortality figures from certain procedures. Although these items may reflect quality of care, they are not true measures of the results of patient care/ outcomes or quality. In addition, data contained in the reports cannot be adjusted by severity of illness or age, sex, income, occupation, or other demographic factors, which further limit comparison between and among plans.

Benefits—Report card information has numerous potential benefits for a variety of audiences:

(1) Employers: to select plans, and assess value of the plan (cost and quality), provide employees information about their benefits, and compare data from plans and make informed decisions about plans that keep their employees healthy and working.

(2) Individual providers: to review performance data prior to contracting with specific health plans as a provider. Report cards that include information regarding a plan's utilization review, and reimbursement and referral patterns (which could affect the provision of care and the individual practitioner's practice style) could help the provider make an informed decision prior to affiliating with a plan.

(3) Administrators, providers, and researchers: to provide valuable information for quality improvement activities and clinical research, to measure a plan's performance and to compare performance with competitors, and to evaluate clinical practice.

(4) Consumers: to select plans that meet individual needs.

Health Plan Employer Data and Information Set (HEDIS)—Report cards range in size and complexity from one-page summaries to two-volume reports covering over 100 performance measures. Some appear to be little more than marketing tools, and most do not allow comparisons to be made among health plans. Continued questions about the integrity of the report cards led to the industry's development of a tool and measurement system for auditing the performance of health plans.

The first work to produce HEDIS 1.0 dates back to the end of the 1980s and early 1990s. HEDIS is a set of performance measures intended for use in evaluating how well a health plan meets the needs of its enrolled population. The primary goal of HEDIS was to standardize the way health plans report information to external audiences, such as purchasers and employers. In this way, it could be more meaningful and comparable across health plans. A related goal was to streamline the reporting process and make it more efficient for the health plan. The initial efforts involved a group of employers and health plans. Since then subsequent versions of HEDIS (2.0 and 2.5) have been produced under the auspices of the National Committee for Quality Assurance, the organization that accredits HMOs. HEDIS evaluates health plans in five major areas of performance:

▼ Quality—how well the plan is doing in providing selected services in four major areas (preventive services, prenatal care, acute and chronic diseases, mental health);

▼ Access and patient satisfaction—how easy it is for patients to use the services and how happy they are with the results;

▼ Membership and use—how many people pick the plan, how many leave, and how often they use selected services;

▼ Finance—how sound and stable the organization is and what has been happening to premiums; and

▼ Descriptive information on health plan management and activities—information related to provider recredentialing and utilization review that affects enrollees' health, satisfaction, and use of services.

Currently, HEDIS includes only process items and is therefore a measure of the plan itself. HEDIS does not specify the clinical status of patients or whether functional status improved as a result of treatment. The next version of HEDIS (3.0) is expected to address some of these issues. It is envisioned that this version will evaluate how health plans manage patients with chronic illnesses and will include a standardized member satisfaction survey. It hopes to be more applicable to Medicare and Medicaid populations, and address risk-adjustment issues so comparisons can be made between and among plans.

CONCLUSION

The literature and experts in the field clearly support the concept of report cards and encourage continued development. Caution continues to be expressed regarding the limitations of the current indicators and what they are able to measure. Further skepticism exists regarding the accuracy of the data sources. With these warnings in mind, market forces continue to push the use of report cards and patient satisfaction surveys and encourage health plans and their providers to be accountable for the care they provide. Employers and individual consumers want to know the value of what they are purchasing in terms of cost and quality. Report cards are being seen as a tool for achieving this purpose. ▼

REFERENCES

Kenkel, P. J. (Ed.). (1995). *Report cards: What every health care provider needs to know about HEDIS and other performance measures.* Gaithersburg, MD: Aspen Publications.

Sinioris, M. E. (1994). QMHC interview: Janet M. Corrigan, Ph.D. *Quality Management in Health Care, 2*(4), 82–89.

U. S. General Accounting Office. (1994). *Health care reform: "Report cards" are useful but significant issues need to be addressed.* GAO/HEHS-94-219. Washington, DC: GAO.

38

Managed Care Legal Issues

SECTION I.
MANAGED CARE CONTRACTING ISSUES

As managed care continues to expand, OT practitioners and health care facilities will have no other option but to sign contracts with managed care organizations (MCOs). As an OT practitioner, whether you contract through provider networks, through health care facilities, or directly with managed care organizations (MCOs), you should have a firm grasp of your legal options and the risks and responsibilities involved in the contracting process.

Your participation in an MCO contract has the same legal force and obligations as any other contract. It is essential that you know exactly which services you have contracted for, the number and types of patients you will be expected to treat each day, and the management and reporting responsibilities to which you have committed yourself.

When contracting through a health care facility, it is imperative for your health care facility to include OT services in its general MCO contract. As an OT, you can help to ensure that this happens by identifying the facility personnel involved with negotiating contracts with MCOs and educating them on OT services.

This section highlights some of the most important contract provisions and strategies to consider when negotiating with MCOs and is followed by a checklist to be used as a guide in your negotiations. This information is not intended as a substitute for legal advice specifically tailored to individual circumstances. It is recommended that you or your facility consult with an attorney before signing any contract.

INVESTIGATE THE MCO

Before you consider entering into a contract, you should investigate the MCO through information obtained from the MCO as well as from independent resources. Talk to other providers and patients associated with the plan, as well as outside agencies responsible for monitoring the plan, such as state regulatory agencies, insurance commissions, and credentialing organizations. Understand who owns the MCO and its corporate structure, its duration in the market, and its financial and credentialing status.

Investigate patient satisfaction with the plan, including disenrollment rates and the frequency of patient change from one provider to another. Get a sense of the plan's reputation for operating appropriate utilization review practices, and investigate the number and types of adverse actions taken against the plan by consumers, providers, and regulatory agencies.

Review the preferred provider list and the facilities included in the MCO. Research the characteristics of the patients this MCO insures, by age, disability, types of services they require, and extent of service utilization over the past several years. Finally, and most important, explore the use of OT and related therapy services, patient therapy needs, utilization and duration of therapy, and the ratio of therapists to patients.

PROFESSIONAL LIABILITY CONCERNS

Define your relationship with the MCO: Your relationship with the MCO has direct bearing on your professional risk of liability. You need to determine whether this contractual relationship will create new types of liability for you that you did not have prior to entering this contract.

A contract should be explicit about the risks and liabilities of both the provider and the MCO. The purpose of hold harmless or indemnification provisions in a contract is to protect against risks and liabilities created by, or arising from, the contractual relationship. MCOs typically require providers to sign contracts containing such provisions, holding the MCO harmless for liabilities that may arise as a result of the provider's conduct. The provider will want to be clear about what specific conduct these provisions apply to. For example, the more controls the primary care physician has over the utilization review/gatekeeping process and determining the need and duration of occupational therapy services, the more the OT's liability should be limited.

Negotiating a mutual indemnification with an MCO may be a reasonable compromise, where the MCO is required to hold the provider harmless for liabilities that may arise as a result of the MCO's conduct, i.e., negligent utilization standards, or negligent selection of providers. **Medical malpractice or professional liability insurance carriers** often object to hold harmless and mutual obligation clauses. Consult with your carrier before signing. Hold harmless clauses can transfer legal responsibilities that may not be acceptable to your insurance carrier or yourself.

If you perform any administration functions for the MCO, make sure the MCO insures you to administer those functions, and determine whether your insurance will protect you if you indemnify for these functions.

There may be other parties to the contract. **It is important that all parties to the contract are clearly defined and that the relationships between these parties are clearly described in the contract.** Your liabilities and responsibilities can vary depending on the type and number of organizations who are party to the contract. For example, your contract may be with a physician-hospital organization that then contracts with a health maintenance organization. Respective roles and responsibilities of every party must be clearly defined.

Similarly, an MCO with whom you contract may offer several "product lines." For example, an MCO may have both an health maintenance organization and a preferred provider organization product line. Your contract should specify your obligations to each product line and how your obligations to future product lines will be handled. Ideally, you will want flexibility to accept or reject each product line. At the very least, details of each should be specified.

The contract should be clear about your continuing liability if you are terminated from the plan, or when the patient is no longer enrolled by the MCO but still requires therapy. The contract should specify whether the MCO's providers are required to cooperate in the mutual defense of a claim.

41

PROFESSIONAL QUALIFICATIONS AND PERFORMANCE

Provider eligibility criteria: In addition to meeting state regulation requirements, such as professional licensure or certification, MCOs are developing their own selection criteria that providers must meet to qualify for participation in the MCO. These requirements may include additional training or may, for example, look at the provider's affiliation with other providers. **Know who is making these qualification decisions for the MCO and what they know about occupational therapy services.** As an initial step, the MCO may require you to complete an application, the contents of which will be made a part of the contract. Also know whether the contract refers to a credentialing manual that describes the application and evaluation process where additional criteria also may be specified.

The MCO will likely have a system for tracking your clinical and financial performance. Research this, and find out what your obligations are for providing documentation. Become familiar with all quality review and improvement procedures.

Provider due process: Know whether the MCO has a grievance process available for decisions made regarding your performance, prior to imposing a corrective action. The contract should specify the corrective actions the MCO can take against you. These can range from termination, requirements for further education or training, compensation changes, clinical privilege restrictions, and withholding or limiting patient referrals.

One very important aspect of the contract terms with an MCO is **exclusivity.** Be aware of MCO contract clauses requiring you to contract with their plan exclusively. Unless you have determined that this arrangement can guarantee you enough patient volume, and based on your initial assessment that this MCO is a good risk, you want to avoid dependency on only one MCO contract.

> A key focus of the managed care contract is the payment method.

Recordkeeping: Make sure the contract is clear about your recordkeeping responsibilities and the ability of the MCO to inspect your records and perform audits.

UTILIZATION MANAGEMENT

Study the MCO's utilization management process. Understand the techniques and criteria for: 1) prior authorization/precertification review including preadmission, special requirements for certain procedures, procedures for specialty care, elective care, and ancillary care; 2) concurrent review; 3) case management; 4) recertification review; 5) prospective/retrospective review; 6) and gatekeeping. Know who specifically performs utilization reviews, i.e., medical director, other medically-trained or nonmedical trained staff, and the specific information involved, paperwork, phone calls, and meetings.

Know who issues denial notices, what specific information is provided, whether an appeal process is available to you to contest a denial on behalf of an enrollee, and **whether you have an obligation to appeal a decision with which you disagree.** A growing number of legal cases have found that a provider's claim that it was following the utilization review orders of the MCO does not necessarily offer the provider legal protection. Courts have held that in addition to the MCO, the provider also has an obligation to act in a patient's best interest by appealing decisions with which it disagrees. **It is important to clearly document your recommended prognosis and plan of treatment.**

The contract should specify what clinical practice guidelines, protocols, pathways, parameters, or other explicit statements that affect approved utilization you are required to follow. The source of these guidelines also should be specified.

42

The contract may contain **"gag" clauses** that impose limits on the type of information providers can offer to their patients. Such clauses can vary in scope, from forbidding providers from discussing alternative treatments with patients not offered by the MCO, to discussing other aspects of the MCO's operation, including grievance procedures available to patients. Such clauses are generally extended to provider's interaction with the public and media or any other situations relating to the MCO's operation. As with utilization review decisions, claiming you were honoring the specifics of the contract by withholding information may not necessarily offer you legal protection. Such clauses have recently come under greater scrutiny by policymakers, with an increasing number of states considering legislation forbidding such clauses in MCO contracts.

FINANCIAL CONCERNS

A key focus of the managed care contract is the payment method. Most MCOs use either a **discounted fee-for-service (FFS) or capitation approach,** but many hybrids of these two structures have developed over time. It is important that you understand the specifics of each payment method for each MCO with which you contract.

Capitation is the method by which the provider receives a fixed payment per enrollee, per period of time, in exchange for providing specified services over a specified period of time. Capitated contracts are preferred by MCOs because they allow the MCO to shift to the provider the risk of furnishing an above-average level of services and to budget more effectively through the ability to predict health care expenses.

43

Requiring the provider to assume risk through "risk withholds" are commonly required by managed care as part of the contract agreements with providers. In these situations, providers are paid only a certain percentage of the agreed upon fees, while the remaining is withheld until the provider meets cost containment or utilization goals of the MCO. To assess the reasonableness of a particular MCO's withhold plan, you need to determine whether the utilization goals are reasonable. Once final terms are agreed to, the key to financial viability is effective case and utilization management.

Increasingly, MCOs are tying hospital, physician and other provider goals together through shared risk pools. **Withhold/risk pools** are funded by an MCO's deduction from each participating provider's payment. You should inquire about these withhold pools. The method for determining the risk pool budget and for sharing risks and rewards among providers who are part of the risk pool should be described in the contract. You should be careful to participate only in pools that include other providers whom you expect will manage their utilization in an appropriate manner.

Stop loss protection should be included in your contract. Stop loss protects the provider against unanticipated losses incurred as a result of high cost cases or unusual large volumes. Stop loss can take the form of per case, per enrollee, or aggregate limitations when the charges for a patient with a particular diagnosis exceed a set dollar threshold. When the threshold is reached, the provider is paid a new reimbursement rate.

Is the reimbursement amount reasonable? Obviously, a threshold item to negotiate in the contract is the FFS or capitation rate. This requires an economic analysis of your practice or facility.

Capitation arrangements should only be entered into where there is a reasonably predictable volume of enrollees during the contractor's applicable term. For a capitation arrangement, the contract should address payment adjustments for increased rates of referrals. For example, the contract could specify that if referrals increase by a certain percentage, the fee should increase by the same percentage.

MCO changing payment levels: It is important that you have some control over the MCO's ability to change payment levels. Your contract should address the circumstances under which changes can be made. An automatic annual increase should be written into the contract to correspond with Consumer Price Index (CPI) increases (or other index of health or medical inflation). In an FFS arrangement, understand what is covered in your fee, i.e., actual therapy time, administrative costs, utilization management responsibilities, and consultation.

Timing of payment and billing requirements: The contract should clearly state how claims are processed and how and when the provider gets paid. The contract will likely require "timely and complete" submission of forms. Understand the consequences if you do not adhere to these requirements, and make sure you use the proper billing codes. The contract should also address late payment penalties for the MCO if it does not pay you on time. Make sure there is a method for dispute resolution if the MCO denies payment. Understand the MCO's rights regarding access to your billing records.

Relationship among various payers: Many contracts contain "no pursuit of payment clauses" prohibiting the provider from pursuing the patient for unpaid bills. The contract should address the relationship between primary and secondary insurance coverage, including your right to pursue payment from other insurance coverage. When other coverage is available and primary, will another plan supplement payment in any way? Can the provider charge a secondary insurer for noncovered services? The contract should specify who is responsible for billing or coordinating secondary insurance, and who is entitled to receipts.

44

TERMINATION

Understand and negotiate under what circumstances your contract can be terminated. **Termination with cause:** the contract should express what is "cause" for termination and the notice period for such termination. Make sure you are not assuming risk for things you have little control over, e.g., meeting utilization guidelines with a complicated case mix. Be clear whether a "breach" automatically terminates the contract and who decides whether there has been a breach, and whether you are given written notice of a breach and a time for cure. A "breach" could occur for violation of any provision in the contract, as well as for other specified problems, e.g., loss of license or loss of malpractice insurance. Termination for cause should be permitted by either party.

Termination without cause: The contract should clearly describe the circumstances under which the contract can be terminated by the MCO without cause. **Due process, the right to appeal such termination** should be negotiated by the provider and expressly stated in the contract. Also, the provider should negotiate the ability to terminate without cause. You want to be able to get out of the contract if the arrangement is not working. Negotiations will not be easy MCOs want the upper hand in termination activity.

Contracts typically contain **"severability"** clauses combined with "change of law" provisions that can substantively affect the terms and termination provisions of the contract. Under severability, if one clause of the contract is illegal or unenforceable, the rest of the contract remains enforceable. **"Change of law" provisions require the parties to renegotiate or reform certain aspects of the contract** that may be changed as a result of changes in laws, regulations, or court interpretations.

Continuity of care: Understand your obligations to patients once you have been terminated, and make sure you can continue to treat patients and be paid until a patient is appropriately referred to another OT practitioner in the MCO plan.

Contract renewal: If you participate in several MCOs, it is advisable to have varying renewal dates and terms of contracts. Agree on contract renewal procedures and understand what terms are renegotiable at the end of the contract term.

Before you sign any agreement, read all documents referenced in the contract, including all policy and procedure memos and all manuals, including the general provider manual and credentialing manuals. The contract should include a definition section—a standard set of definitions should be adopted for the entire set of documents. If the MCO can amend policies and procedures found in these documents, these changes should be limited to non-substantive changes. The operational and clinical policies and procedures can vary greatly from one MCO to another. *Review all aspects of the MCO agreement thoroughly with assistance from a lawyer who practices in the area of health law.*

CHECKLIST FOR CONTRACTING WITH AN MCO

Investigate the MCO

▼ Who owns the MCO, and what is the MCO's corporate structure?

▼ What is the MCO's financial and credentialing status?

▼ How long has the MCO been operating?

Documentation and Definitions

▼ How many different documents exists describing MCO policies and procedures?

▼ Does the MCO have a standard set of definitions for the entire set of documents?

Scope of Services/Providers

▼ What health care services and items are covered by the MCO? How are coverage and exclusions described?

▼ What is the utilization of OT services? What level of referrals or volumes of service can the OT expect?

▼ What types and numbers of providers are included on the preferred provider list? What is the ratio of providers to enrollees? What and who determines when more providers will be added?

▼ Does the MCO or a regulatory agency have information available to review on patient satisfaction, enrollment and disenrollment rates, services utilization, outcomes data, etc.?

Professional Liability Concerns

▼ Is the contract explicit about the risks and liabilities of both the provider and the MCO?

▼ Does the contract include a hold harmless or indemnification provision requiring the provider to indemnify the MCO for claims by enrollees? Is the contract clear about what specific conduct this applies to?

▼ Does the contract also indemnify the provider for liabilities that may arise as a result of the MCO's conduct?

- ▼ Does the contract specify the provider's obligations to each of the "product lines" (i.e., PPO, HMO) of the MCO?

- ▼ What is the provider's continuing liability if terminated from a plan?

- ▼ Does the contract require the provider to contract with this MCO exclusively?

Professional Qualifications and Performance

- ▼ What are the MCO's selection criteria for providers?

- ▼ Who is making these qualification decisions, and what do they know about OT?

- ▼ Is the provider required to complete an application that becomes part of the contract?

- ▼ Does the contract refer to a credentialing manual that describes the application and evaluation process?

- ▼ How does the MCO track the provider's clinical and financial performance? What are the provider's obligations for providing documentation for this process? Does the MCO have access to the provider's clinical and financial records?

- ▼ Does the MCO have a grievance process available for decisions made regarding the provider's performance?

Utilization Management

- ▼ What is the MCO's process for making decisions regarding an enrollee's access to care? Are the decision makers clearly defined?

- ▼ Does the contract or other documentation specify the criteria and eligibility for:

   (a) precertification review, including access to specialty care, elective care, experimental care, emergency care, and ancillary care

   (b) concurrent review

   (c) case management

   (d) recertification review

   (e) retrospective review?

- ▼ How is this information recorded and confirmed?

- ▼ Does the contract specify the clinical practice guidelines, protocols, pathways, parameters, or other explicit guidelines that should be used in making care decisions?

- ▼ Can pre-admission or referral approval be rescinded retroactively?

- ▼ Can enrollees seek care from providers outside of the MCO's network of providers? Under what circumstances?

- ▼ Is there an appeals process available to both the enrollee and the provider to contest a denial of care?

- ▼ Does the contract contain "gag" clauses imposing limits on the type of information providers can provide to enrollees?

Financial Concerns

- ▼ What payment method is used in the contract?

- ▼ Does the contract require the provider to assume risk through "risk withholds" that reasonably relate to the MCO's utilization goals?

- ▼ Does the contract contain stop loss protection?

- ▼ Is the reimbursement amount reasonable?

- ▼ Does the contract address the circumstances under which the MCO can change payment levels? Does the MCO automatically adjust payment levels annually? If a capitated method is used, does the contract address payment adjustments for increased rates of referral?

- ▼ What are the terms and time lines for processing payment claims? What are the provider's responsibilities? What coding method is used? Does the contract address late payment penalties for the MCO if it does not pay the provider on time? Does the MCO have access to the provider's billing records? Is there a method for resolving payment disputes?

- ▼ Does the contract address the relationship between primary and secondary insurance coverage and whether the provider can pursue other payment sources, including the enrollee, for unpaid bills?

Termination

- ▼ Does a "breach" automatically terminate the contract, and who decides whether there has been a breach? Are all conditions under which a breach can occur specified in the contract? Does the contract require written notice of a breach and a time for cure?

- ▼ Does the contract clearly describe the circumstances under which the contract can be terminated without cause? Does the provider have the right to appeal such termination?

- ▼ Does the provider have a right to terminate the contract?

- ▼ If terminated, what are the MCO's continuing obligations to pay for services, or the provider's obligation to continue providing care, midstream in a course of treatment?

- ▼ What are the terms for contract renewal? Is the contract automatically renewed? What terms are renegotiable? Does the contract continue during renewal negotiations?

II. JOINING OR FORMING A NETWORK

Occupational therapy practitioners need to be active in assessing their options for assuring their place in the new and competitive era of managed care. To remain competitive, independent practicing OTs need to consider associating with larger networks of providers. Collectively, providers have more leverage in marketing their services to MCOs. Increasingly, MCOs are abandoning discounted fee-for-service negotiations with individual practitioners and are interested in contracting only through larger networks using capitation and other methods of assuming risk by networks.

Associating with a network can be beneficial. As MCOs place new demands on providers to become more efficient and more cost effective, many providers are finding it useful to join larger networks. By combining efforts, these providers are more effectively establishing systems for demonstrating clinical outcomes and maintaining patient satisfaction data, as well as operating more cost efficient practices and saving time and management costs for both their practices and the MCO with which they are contracting.

Your ultimate goal in forming or joining a network should be to maximize your business interests. You will still continue operating your own practice. You may choose to affiliate with several networks.

Critical factors to consider in forming and joining any network include **tax consequences of the corporate structure of the network, the liability of the network's owners, the ability or necessity for the network to raise capital, the overall governance of the network, and adherence to antitrust rules.**

Several **corporate structures** are available to providers, depending on the goals and concerns of their network. For example, a C-corporation and a limited liability company (not available in every state) should be considered to protect the owners from unlimited liability where there is a potential for malpractice or other liability. Better arrangements exists if the primary goal is to make a profit at the network level. In this case, a partnership should be used to avoid taxes at the entity level. You should consult an attorney who specializes in corporate law for assistance in identifying the range of potential corporate structures and in determining the corporate structure that bests meets your goals.

Many of the risks involved with operating and participating in a network depend on the type of corporate structure, particularly with regard to professional liability risks. You may be at risk for joint liability, the ability to hold all network providers responsible for the negligence of one provider. Suits brought by providers not included in the network are also a possibility. Business risks associated with starting or investing in any business should be analyzed. You should carefully examine the liability and business risks of associating with a network by consulting an attorney who practices in this area.

Determining the **governance structure** involves identifying and/or establishing the role and authority of the various providers associated with the network. The network plan should identify an administrative structure and determine voting rights of network members. The corporate structure chosen will help to define the governance options available to the network. If you are joining an already established network, you want to examine the governance structure closely to determine whether your interests are represented in the decision making process, i.e., whether OTs are in decision-making positions and whether there is an equal distribution across provider types and specialties in all decision-making situations, including administrative positions, boards of directors, and planning committees. If you are establishing a network, you also want to consider representation across all provider types and specialties who you want to encourage to participate in the network.

Reviewing all documentation associated with the network is critical. Included among these documents are articles of incorporation, bylaws, shareholder agreements, participating provider agreements, provider credentialing standards, and MCO contracts. By becoming active in the governing structure of the network, you may have an opportunity to participate in the drafting of some of these documents. Also, you should ask about network membership fees.

One example of a network organized by an OT and a PT is the New England Therapy Network (NET) Limited Liability Co. in Connecticut. NET is a multidisciplinary network of OT, PT, speech/language pathology, medical social work, vocational counseling, and audiology. Organizers of this network are marketing their ability to save MCOs money by managing the rehabilitation component in a quality, cost-conscious way. NET expects to reduce administrative costs through centralized insurance authorization and electronic billing and collections, and it is contemplating hiring a management firm. The network's recruiting procedures involve committee credentialing of both facilities and therapists. There are similar networks in several states, including California, Texas, Arizona, Minnesota, New York, New Jersey, and Illinois.

Antitrust Implications of Networks

Any network affiliation must be carefully structured to avoid a potential violation of many laws and regulations, including antitrust laws.

Collective action by independently practicing providers in determining fees or deciding whether to contract with an MCO can result in antitrust violations. A key reason to rely on a formal network structure is to ensure you are complying with antitrust laws as you join together with other OT practices to compete for MCO contracts.

> It is important that you identify how your network meets economic integration requirements.

Antitrust laws prohibit any concerted action that unreasonably restrains competition and creates monopolies in the marketplace. Concerted action is the association of competing entities. The integration or joining of formerly competitive entities into a new organizational structure raises antitrust concerns.

51

The U. S. Department of Justice (DOJ) and the Federal Trade Commission (FTC) enforce the federal antitrust laws. DOJ and FTC jointly issued two sets of guidelines in September 1993 and September 1994 *(DOJ and FTC, Statements of Antitrust Enforcement Policy in the Health Care Area, 4 Trade Reg. Rep. (CCH) 13,151, September 15, 1993; DOJ and FTC, Statements of Enforcement Policy and Analytical Principles Relating to Health Care and Antitrust, 4 Trade Reg. Rep. (CCH) 13,152, September 27, 1994)* to assist providers in understanding antitrust laws pertaining to a range of health care activities including organizing networks. These guidelines explain the process the agencies will use in determining whether a particular network violates the antitrust laws.

Under the antitrust laws, most conduct is examined under a **"rule of reason"** analysis. However, some types of conduct are considered always to be anticompetitive. These types of conduct are said to be **"per se"** illegal, regardless of their purpose or actual effect on competition. **Price-fixing agreements and group boycotts are per se illegal.** An agreement among competing providers to request particular fee levels from MCOs is price fixing. Any evidence of price tampering is highly suspect. An agreement among competing providers to jointly refuse to deal with an MCO is a group boycott.

To avoid violations of the antitrust laws, OTs need to know how they can **"integrate"** their practices with the effect of reducing antitrust risk when engaged in collective negotiations with payers. Integration requires substantial sharing of economic risk.

Fully integrated networks in which providers entirely merge two or more practices into one practice are considered to be single entities for antitrust purposes and therefore not subject to concerted action concerns. In most cases, however, the networks that OTs are considering joining are likely only **partially integrated.** In these situation, OTs who will remain competitors for some purposes will form a network to practice more efficiently or to offer a service that they could not offer as effectively without the network. Networks of this nature involve **partial integration.**

It is important that you identify how your network meets economic integration requirements. You need to show **financial risk sharing and/or the creation of efficiencies.** Examples of situations that have satisfied economic integration requirements include:

- ▼ significant capital from providers to establish the network,

- ▼ risk sharing through a capitation reimbursement mechanism or a significant fee withhold,

- ▼ consolidating business functions, such as administration, claims processing, billing, personnel, purchasing and marketing,

- ▼ establishment of peer review, utilization management, case management, and quality assurance mechanisms.

The greater the degree of integration, the less likely the network will be subject to antitrust scrutiny.

Having determined there is sufficient economic integration, a "rule of reason" analysis is applied. This involves defining the relevant market and evaluating the procompetitive effects and efficiencies of the network.

Partially integrated networks cannot include too large a percentage of competing providers in the relevant market for risk of creating a monopoly of those providers. The **relevant market** examined includes both the **relevant services market and the relevant geographic market. The relevant services market** is defined as the array of services these providers compete to provide—this market will likely include several specialties that compete with each other to provide the same or very similar services. **The relevant geographic market** is defined as broad enough to include all providers viewed by insurance payers as good substitutes for the providers in the network.

If a high proportion of OTs (and similar competitive providers) integrate into a network, there is antitrust risk that the affiliation could hinder or blockade vigorous competition among other OTs (and similar competitive providers). This concern might arise, for example, if an MCO could not recruit a viable panel of participating OTs (and other similar providers) without contracting with this network.

Evaluating the competitive effects of the network involves determining whether the network has a large percentage of the relevant market to enable it to exclude other similar ventures from the relevant market. If a sufficient number of similar networks exists, or if a large number of OTs (or similar competitive providers) are available to form similar networks, it is unlikely that the network has anticompetitive effects. This is especially true when the network is non-exclusive, permitting its members to participate in other networks or similar ventures.

Evaluating the procompetitive efficiencies involves assessing the potential of the network to create efficiencies through the administrative procedures, utilization review mechanisms, quality assurance programs, and similar mechanisms.

Negotiating payment with MCOs: a critical antitrust requirement for partially integrated networks is that each network member make his or her own independent decisions about price. The collective provision of fee information is subject to substantial antitrust risk. The network can serve as an effective negotiating agent for participating providers as long as important antitrust rules are followed. Antitrust case law has defined acceptable procedures for price negotiations with health insurance payers. Under the **"strict messenger model,"** the network employs a neutral third-party agent to solicit contracts and receive offers from payers, presenting these offers to each network provider individually. Each provider must respond independently to whether he or she is willing to accept the payer's prices and participate under such an offer.

In the past, variations to the messenger model have been acceptable to antitrust authorities for network negotiations with payers, but more recently, these alternatives have come under greater scrutiny.

MULTIPROVIDER NETWORKS

Escalation of managed care in the health care market place has also resulted in hospitals, physicians, and others providers coming together to organize their own managed care plans to compete with the health insurance companies. An increasing number of these providers are exercising their option in forming **multiprovider networks** to provide a full range of affordable, quality services. These new entities, commonly referred to as *provider* (or *physi-*

cian)-hospital organizations (PHOs, or provider service networks/PSNs, or provider service organizations/PSOs) are creating new challenges for antitrust regulators as they evaluate the **"integration"** issues related to these structures.

The threshold antitrust issue for PHOs is the extent of economic integration. Antitrust guidelines require PHOs to offer only products that put ***all*** PHO participants at substantial financial risk (i.e., capitation or significant fee withholds) or use the strict messenger model in price negotiations.

Antitrust laws have been used to challenge MCO action in **excluding or refusing to admit certain providers** in their plans. In the past, case law has tended to favor the MCO in exclusionary actions, with antitrust authorities more concerned with over-inclusion and creating monopolies rather than selectivity of providers. Refusal to admit, or a decision to terminate, a provider from a plan could be viewed as a concerted refusal to deal by the provider members. An MCO's defense under such a claim can be that certain providers do not meet cost containment standards and thus will not enhance efficiency or pro-competitive goals. The fundamental focus of these types of cases will be the impact of the MCO's actions on overall competition in the relevant market.

Some states also have their own antitrust laws enforced by the state attorney general. Several states have moved to override federal antitrust laws under certain conditions operating under a doctrine known as **"state action immunity."** These laws have been primarily aimed at helping hospitals, physician, and other providers in forming integrated multi-provider networks and with hospital mergers.

Application of antitrust law to the variety of health care networks forming to compete in the changing health care market is very complicated and fact intensive. ***Seek advice from attorneys knowledgeable in health antitrust law before forming or joining networks.***

III. STATE LAWS GOVERNING MANAGED CARE

As managed care continues to expand as a way to control health care costs, questions have arisen regarding restrictions of consumer choice of provider, access to necessary care, and compromised quality of care. An increasing number of states are responding to these concerns by regulating various aspects of managed care operations. Theses laws vary greatly from state to state, both in types of managed care issues addressed and in the intensity of oversight of managed care plans.

Included among these state laws are mandates requiring coverage of certain health care services and coverage of these services by certain providers, mandates addressing provider selection for MCO participation, patient access and quality of care standards for MCOs including requirements that patients can seek care outside of an MCO network, and requirements concerning information disclosure to patients and regulations addressing utilization review practices. So called "any willing provider" and "freedom of choice" laws have been making their way through state legislatures for some time, as have laws mandating certain health care benefits. More recently, several states have passed or are considering "omnibus" bills that address a range of "consumer and provider protection" issues with regard to MCO participation.

It is important to understand the distinctions between the various issues these laws seek to address. Explanation of these laws will often consolidate many of these provisions into convenient umbrella descriptions, for example, some descriptions of "any willing provider" laws have combined a range of laws regulating provider participation in MCOs. Not surprisingly, MCOs generally do not favor regulating any aspect of managed care and generally describe many of these efforts as "anti-managed care," concerned that any regulation interferes with cost control mechanisms and their ability to "manage" care.

REGULATING PROVIDER PARTICIPATION IN MCOS

Any willing provider laws require MCOs to include *every* provider, who meets the terms and conditions of the health plan, as a participant in the plan. At first glance, this language appears to allow any provider to participate in an MCO, but the "reach" of such laws varies greatly from state to state. These laws may limit the **types of providers** qualified to take advantage of this law by defining qualified "providers" narrowly in the law. The law will include a definition section naming specific types of providers who qualify, or will state the intent to include all providers who are **authorized by state law to provide "covered" services.** Many states have passed any willing provider laws that have been restricted to a select group of providers, e.g., hospitals, pharmacists, and chiropractors. Similarly, these laws have varied in the types of health plans that are subject to these laws, e.g., HMOs and PPOs. Finally, the MCO's "terms and conditions" that must be met by these providers may be restrictive so as to disqualify otherwise qualified providers. MCOs are concerned that any willing provider laws constrain their ability to limit the number of providers and to select only cost-effective providers for their panels.

Freedom-of-choice laws require MCOs to reimburse every type of provider who is licensed to provide "covered" services, for the services they render. Generally these laws are written to recognize all types of providers who are authorized by state law to provide covered services. These laws may vary in the types of health plans subject to these provisions. These laws are particularly directed at situations where an individual chooses to go out-of-network to seek care from a different type of licensed provider than those included on the MCO's panel of network providers.

Antidiscrimination provisions prohibit MCOs from arbitrarily excluding entire classes or types of licensed professionals from their provider network panels. Under these laws, MCOs are forbidden from discriminating against professionals based on the type of license (or certification or registration) the professional holds. AOTA has actively supported these provisions as a reasonable alternative to any willing provider laws because they ensure that MCOs will have a range of qualified health professionals available to consumers while also recognizing the legitimate interests of MCOs to limit the number of providers and to control costs.

Some MCOs have not included OTs among their network of rehabilitation providers. In some cases this is intentional, deciding only to use other types of providers. In other cases, it is conceivable that the MCO is not familiar with OT as a separate and distinct licensed profession. One example of discrimination might involve the MCO's preapproval of hand therapy where an OT may find himself or herself in a situation where, because the plan only recognizes licensed physical therapists, he or she may be denied payment once the therapy has been provided. You should become familiar with the list of providers and covered services for each MCO, and educate the MCO on your profession and the range of services you are qualified to provide.

State laws and bills that have prohibited discrimination based on licensure generally have specified other conditions of participation and have imposed other measures that allow MCOs to control costs. As long as these conditions are applied evenly across providers, state laws have allowed MCOs to:

▼ limit the number and types of providers,

▼ use geographic areas, low utilization rates, and range of provider services as non-discriminatory selection criteria,

▼ exclude groups of specialized providers by utilizing an economic rationale,

▼ discriminate "reasonably" against providers by limiting their panel, as long as the network effectively reduces health care costs, and

▼ rely on a provider's willingness to abide by management and UR requirements as a selection criterion.

In the case of institutional providers, case law has allowed price differences among otherwise equally qualified providers to be acceptable economic rationale for choosing one provider over another, even in the situation where, because of geographic location, one provider had to charge more than the other. Generally, unless state laws impose additional quality care standards, MCOs have broad discretion in demonstrating that their provider selection criteria meet economic goals.

While antidiscrimination laws, and similar provider participation laws, do not guarantee that you will be included in MCO network panels, these laws are a major step toward requiring MCOs to use specific selection criteria and to explain this criteria to health care professionals who apply to participate in the MCO's plan.

Provider due process laws require MCOs to follow certain procedures in creating and maintaining networks of providers, such as publishing the criteria for participation in the network and providing for an appeal process in the event of termination of a provider from participation in the network. These provisions generally are found in laws that address a range of regulations pertaining to MCO operations.

Regulation of provider participation in MCOs is a growing and evolving area of law. So far, however, legal action brought under state laws, primarily under any willing provider laws, and primarily by institutional providers, has favored the MCO. These cases can shed some light on the evaluation process MCOs should follow in selecting providers to avoid a legal challenge. These cases have allowed MCOs to restrict provider membership in a network as long as such restriction is exercised reasonably. This requires a "thorough comparative analysis" of the providers in the targeted geographic area and calculation of the cost efficiency of each provider. Application of these criterion to individual health professionals will pose additional challenges for MCOs.

REGULATING CONSUMER PROTECTIONS

State laws addressing **access standards for MCOs** authorize the insurance commissioner or other state authority to oversee and promulgate regulations requiring MCOs to demonstrate that they have the resources and capacity to meet the range of needs of plan enrollees. These provisions may be explicit on a range of requirements including specifying that MCOs:

- ▼ have a sufficient number, mix, and distribution of health professionals in their network panel;

- ▼ ensure covered services are available and accessible in the service area of the plan, through a variety of sites and with reasonable proximity to the residences and workplaces of enrollees;

▼ provide services with reasonable promptness (including reasonable hours of
    operation and after-hours service; and

▼ reasonably assure the continuity of care.

Generally included along with access standards or in separate legislation are **information reporting and disclosure requirements.** Included among theses provisions may be
requirements that the MCO make available to enrollees information regarding benefits
included as well as excluded from the plan, information on the types and distribution of
health providers, including specialists in the plan and excluded from the plan, and the ratio
of enrollees to participating providers. Also included might be a requirement that MCOs
disclose their financial arrangements with providers.

Two alternative approaches have been proposed in state legislation to address an
enrollee's ability to seek health care services outside of an MCO's network. One option is
to require an MCO that offers a closed panel plan (e.g., a staff-model health maintenance
organization) to also offer a **point-of-service** plan. The other option is to require all MCOs,
regardless of their type (e.g., HMO, PPO, IPO, etc.), to allow enrollees to go **out of network** to receive care, applying an additional copayment requirement. Some variations on
this requirement have specified conditions or limited the circumstances under which

enrollees can seek care outside of the MCO network of providers. (The terms *point-of-service*
and *out-of-network* have been used interchangeably to describe these situations.)

Utilization review requirements have been imposed on MCOs by some states to
ensure that these procedures are not only used as mechanisms to control costs, but also to
ensure enrollees have access to all necessary and appropriate care. Among the provisions
addressed are:

▼ disclosure requirements to enrollees regarding clinical guidelines used and the
    names and credentials of decision makers,

▼ requirements addressing the formulation of these guidelines, including the involve-
    ment of appropriately trained medical staff,

▼ the use of non-medically and medically trained staff in making care decisions,

▼ utilization requirements regarding emergency vs. non-emergency care decisions,

▼ the treatment of preauthorization review decisions as final determinations for the
    purpose of making payment,

▼ gatekeeping provisions, including the use of specialists as gatekeepers for enrollees
    with special health care needs or chronic conditions, and

▼ direct access to specialist requirements in certain situations.

On a related issue, an increasing number of states are prohibiting the use of **"gag"** **clauses** in MCO contracts with providers. These clauses restrict what providers may communicate to patients regarding treatment, including alternative treatment/therapies that may be a viable option for the enrollee's health care needs.

More states are addressing the need for allowing enrollees to have some recourse for questioning MCO decisions by requiring MCOs to develop **grievance procedures,** under **consumer due process laws.** These procedures provide a mechanism by which enrollees are informed of MCO decisions regarding access to health care and are offered an opportunity to respond to these decisions, especially when access is denied. Some state laws have required MCOs to develop very comprehensive grievance procedures, providing enrollees with an opportunity to question all health care decisions. In other states, these laws have been more narrow in focus, allowing enrollees to only question emergency care decisions.

State laws have also addressed **benefit mandates** directing MCOs to cover certain health care services and items. The services and items, as well as the type of MCOs covered under these laws, vary across state laws.

This review of state law is not exhaustive of the array of laws states are passing and considering as they grapple with consumers' concerns with the changing health care market and as they seek to define the appropriate level of oversight of this market.

IV. FRAUD AND ABUSE: ANTI-KICKBACK AND SELF-REFERRAL LAWS

Health care fraud and abuse cost the nation an estimated $100 billion in 1995, representing approximately 10 percent of health care spending. Over the past few years, one area of fraud and abuse investigative activity and policy changes has focused on the proliferation of financial relationships that exist between physicians and the other health care providers to whom they refer patients. Concerns have been voiced about the appropriateness of such arrangements and the effects they can have on the decisions made by physicians in determining the services required by their patients.

Physicians have financial interests in a wide array of businesses, including clinical laboratories, radiology facilities, durable medical equipment suppliers, rehabilitation agencies or clinics, nursing homes, and home health care agencies. Typically, these types of arrangements take the form of joint ventures, limited partnerships, and other similar organizational structures. As these various entities position themselves to compete in a managed care marketplace, they are being examined for their ability to lead to a guaranteed referral base for the physicians and other providers involved in these ventures. The legal and ethical concerns that arise from these arrangements relate to the cost of health care, the utilization of care, a patient's choice of care, the delivery of quality care, and competition in the marketplace.

Under the Medicare and Medicaid programs, the anti-kickback statute and the physician self-referral laws are the main laws for combatting fraud and abuse activity. Health care fraud and abuse activity also has been prosecuted under the federal criminal code, utilizing such provisions as the mail and wire fraud statutes.

ANTI-KICKBACK STATUTE

The Medicare/Medicaid **anti-kickback statute,** found in Section 1128(b) of the Social Security Act, **is a broad criminal statute requiring proof of *intentional* offering or payment of anything of value in exchange for the referral of Medicare or Medicaid reimbursed items or services.** Penalties include criminal sanctions as well as exclusion from participation in these two federal health care programs.

The anti-kickback statute is administered by the Office of the Inspector General (OIG) of the U.S. Department of Health and Human Services (HHS) and by the U.S. Department of Justice (DOJ). Both case law and subsequent "safe harbors" have helped define abusive arrangements in several areas of health care practice, including joint ventures and self-referral practices.

In 1989, the OIG issued a *Fraud Alert on Joint Venture Arrangements*, specifying the types of investment arrangements between physicians and providers of ancillary services considered to be in violation of the anti-kickback statute. This alert offered the first explanation that the anti-kickback statute applied to self-referral practices. The OIG also has issued a series of special fraud alerts on a range of health care industry practices, including financial arrangements between hospitals and hospital-based physicians and joint venture arrangements.

Potential illegal activity can arise when physicians as investors refer their patients to these entities in which they have invested and are "paid" by the entity in the form of "profit distributions." The impetus behind forming this joint venture may be less to have capital for the venture and more *to lock up a stream of referrals from the physicians and to compensate them indirectly for these referrals*. In analyzing such arrangements, the OIG examines how investors are selected, whether they are chosen because they are in a position to make referrals, and how their investment shares compare to their level of referrals. The nature of the business structure is investigated to determine whether each party is really fully participating in the venture or rather that a "shell" venture has been created. Financing and profit distributions can provide evidence of the true nature and intent of the joint venture.

The OIG is authorized under the law to promulgate safe harbors. Safe harbors carve out areas of legal conduct. Arrangements that otherwise might be subject to enforcement under the anti-kickback law are protected if they meet the detailed regulatory requirements of one or more safe harbor. The OIG has used this authority narrowly. Several safe harbors address ownership and compensation arrangements between physicians and entities to which they refer. Under investment interests rules, for example, no more than 40 percent of a partnership's business can come from investors.

PHYSICIAN SELF-REFERRAL LAWS

The Medicare and Medicaid **physician self-referral laws** were born out of the belief that patient care should not be affected by the referring physician's financial interest. These laws prohibit a physician from referring patients to a "designated service" in which the physician, or an immediate family member, has an ownership or investment interest or a compensation agreement. Compensation arrangements include salary and consultation payments to the physician (or immediate family member) or when a physician pays the entity for items or services. Such payments can be direct or indirect, overt or covert, in-cash or in-kind. In addition to direct referrals, referrals also can occur when a physician requests another physician's consultation and that physician orders tests and services, or when the physician establishes a plan of care that includes designated services.

The first of these laws (Stark I) prohibited Medicare providers from making referrals to clinical laboratories in which they had ownership or investment interests. The scope of this law was expanded in 1993 (Stark II) to apply to Medicaid and to extend the self-referral prohibition to 10 additional types of services, including: physical therapy services; occupational therapy services; radiology and other diagnostic services; radiation therapy services; durable medical equipment; parenteral and enteral nutrients, equipment and supplies; prosthetics, orthotics and prosthetic devices; home health services; outpatient prescription drugs; and inpatient and outpatient hospital services. These laws are described in Section 1877 of the Social Security Act (42 U.S.C. Section 1395nn).

Unlike the anti-kickback statute that requires the proof of intent, Stark I and II are triggered by the mere fact that a financial relationship exists — it does not matter what the physician intends when he or she makes a referral. Medicare or Medicaid will not pay for a service ordered by a physician who has a financial relationship with the service, unless the relationship fits within one of the many enumerated exceptions. A primary target of physician self-referral laws are traditional joint ventures between physicians and ancillary service facilities —- these types of joint ventures are clearly impermissible.

There are several exceptions to these physician self-referral laws; it is recommended that you consult an attorney to determine whether a particular financial situation qualifies for an exception. Among the exceptions related to both ownership/investment and compensation arrangements are physicians' services when a physician refers to a member of the same legitimate **group practice,** certain **in-office ancillary services** furnished by solo practitioners, and group practices and services furnished by certain organizations with **prepaid plans** (i.e., some HMOs). Among the exceptions pertaining only to ownership/investment arrangements are designated services furnished by a **rural provider.** Compensation arrangement exceptions address such situations as payments for the rental of office space and equipment, and **hospital payment relationships with physicians.** Each exception contains specific enumerated requirements that must be met to qualify for an exemption. HCFA has issued regulations on Stark I but not Stark II.

JOINT VENTURES AND INTEGRATED DELIVERY SYSTEMS

MCOs are concerned that anti-kickback and physician self-referral laws interfere with compensation and care delivery arrangements designed by MCOs to save money. Creating new, broad exceptions for managed care in fraud and abuse policies is difficult because the term managed care is not well-defined. Application of these laws to vertically integrated delivery systems that include hospitals, physicians, and other providers, create new challenges in determining how hospitals and physicians and other providers should interact. In these structures, it is important to be aware of an attempt to disguise inappropriate economic gain under the claim of efficient use of health care dollars. Some managed care situations, like HMOs, typically operate as prepaid plans where conditions of participation and rules of financing are well defined. HMOs typically remove physicians from financial incentives to refer patients to other ancillary services. In other cases, such as preferred provider organization arrangements, where the structure is only partially integrated and discounted fee-for-service payments are used, physicians and ancillary service providers may agree to accept a lower price for their services, but these PPO physicians also may be owners of a rehabilitation service center that is part of the PPO network and gain profits from referring patients to this entity.

While HCFA fraud alerts in the area of joint ventures have primarily addressed potential legal liability arrangements involving physicians and hospitals, other types of providers may find themselves in similar situations. **Many of these situations involve both the anti-kickback statute and the physician self-referral laws.**

Violations in these relationships have involved remunerations inconsistent with the fair market value where one party to the agreement is really compensating the other party for expected referrals. For example, HCFA addresses the situation where physicians provide payments or remuneration to hospitals in excess of the fair market value of the services provided by them. Highly suspect as violations of the anti-kickback statute, examples of these arrangements include: physicians paying a portion of their cash receipts in excess of a predetermined amount to the hospital, or a hospital providing no payment to physicians for their services under Part A Medicare in exchange for the physicians' opportunity to perform Part B services.

Purchasing their "flow of business" or "locking up the referral stream" of a physician practice, involves the hospital purchasing a provider's practice or a clinic operation when the hospital is really interested in the future flow of business. **It is illegal under the anti-kickback statute to pay providers now for the flow of business expected in the future.** HCFA has said that this same concern can arise when another entity purchases a physician's practice, if this same entity also owns or operates a hospital that benefits from referrals from the physician.

The payment of bonuses to providers who are employees or independent contractors with a hospital is another area of concern. Typical violations have involved hospitals' **sharing a percentage of the revenue from ancillary services with referring physicians.** A fully capitated payment system mitigates this concern, because hospitals would not be paying incentives for more services; rather the concern here would be underservice. The problem is more of a concern in partially integrated structures, where discounted fee-for-service payments are used.

"**Practice enhancements**" are also a problem, where hospitals offer physicians "incentives" to recruit and retain these physicians. These and similar situations are troubling for their potential interference with the physician's judgment of what is the most appropriate care for the patient, and the ability to inflate costs to the Medicare and Medicaid programs by causing the physician to overutilize inappropriate and unnecessary services. Examples of these incentives include: the use of free or significantly discounted space; payment for a physician's continuing education courses, travel, and conference costs; the provision of free or significantly discounted billing, nursing or other staff services; and agreements to supplement a physician's income if it fails to reach a predetermined level.

HCFA also has addressed kickbacks in exchange for the referral of reimbursable **home health services.** In these situations, home care providers offer kickbacks to physicians, hospitals, and other providers in return for referrals. Kickbacks in these situations have taken the form of payments to a physician for each plan of care certified by the physician, disguis-

63

ing referral fees for salaries as services not rendered, offering free service to beneficiaries like transportation if they switch home care providers, providing hospitals with discharge planners or home care liaisons to induce referrals.

Under the physician self-referral laws, **group practice arrangements with hospitals** that began prior to December 1989 are permissible. These arrangements must adhere to specific requirements, including that the services be billed by the hospital and follow inpatient service guidelines.

The volume or value of future referrals to ancillary services once owned by the physician is also a concern. Violations can occur with extended financing deals where physicians sell their practice or interests in ancillary facilities reflecting an implied understanding that, if they want to get paid, they know they should send their patients to these facilities in the future. The physician self-referral laws require that such a purchase involve a fair market value price, be commercially reasonably, and not be related to the volume or value of referrals. Regarding a sale of practice, under the anti-kickback statute, the sale must be completed within one year, after which the provider/seller can no longer be in a professional position to refer business to the purchasing practitioner.

Under the physician self-referral laws, an exception is made for physician ownership in a hospital, providing the physician has ownership in the entire hospital and not just one division or service area. Salary payments to physicians from hospitals cannot depend on **the volume or value of referrals by the physician to the hospital.** Productivity bonuses are permitted under physician self-referral for hospital employees, as long as these bonuses are based on services personally performed by the physician and not the amount or value of services the physician orders for the hospital. Contracts are permitted between physicians and hospitals for the physician's performance of additional services, such as for consulting services, as long as the contract remuneration does not take into consideration the volume or value of referral services. Hospitals also can hire physicians to run utilization review programs or to oversee the operation of a particular department, as long as the remuneration does not relate to the provision of designated health services.

As you seek opportunities to remain competitive in the health care marketplace by entering into joint venture arrangements with other providers, you should **seek legal advice regarding the application of the anti-kickback and physician self-referral laws to these new arrangements.**

64

OTHER AREAS OF FRAUD AND ABUSE CONCERN

While this section has sought to highlight potential fraud and abuse violations regarding new structures for managed care arrangements, other areas of Medicare and Medicaid fraud and abuse activity have been a focus for policymakers. For example, the operation and billing practices of skilled nursing facilities regarding therapy services were examined in an investigation and report released by the Government Accounting Office (GAO) in 1995 *(GAO Report to the Ranking Minority Member, Committee on Commerce, U.S. House of Representatives: Medicare, Tighter Rules Needed to Curtail Overcharges for Therapy in Nursing Homes, March 1995).* ▼

65

Impact on Facility-Based Delivery of Services

(The following article—while focusing on facility-based service delivery—is also directly applicable to private practice. The two articles that follow, on home health and mental health, address aspects that are different or unique to these areas of service delivery. —Editor)

ORGANIZATIONAL CHANGES

The most obvious effect of the increase in managed care in health care is the demand for services that cost less. This effect has forced health care institutions to take a very hard look at their organization in terms of the cost structure.

Hospital administrators have had to make hard decisions regarding organization charts and staffing in general. The traditional hierarchy has frequently been flattened significantly, putting much more responsibility in the hands of fewer individuals.

Downsizing and *re-engineering* are terms that are often heard when administrators speak of how they are responding to the managed care situation. To lower the cost of providing services in institutions, decreases in staffing numbers across all departments are occurring. This is happening because salary expense is a major part of any facility's operations budget.

Some major goals for facilities in this new environment are to

▼ increase the number of contracts with managed care companies;

▼ increase volume in general (e.g., number of patients seen by the facility, number of visits per month/year);

▼ increase the efficiencies in the delivery of care and, in turn, process and clinical outcomes;

▼ decrease the cost of delivery of care;

▼ offer a competitive price; and

▼ maintain the quality of care.

Managed care companies have some basic criteria and expectations when they are deciding on contracts:

▼ competitive pricing;

▼ availability of network/system of care;

▼ one-stop shopping;

▼ full continuum of care or menu services;

▼ easy access to all parts of the system;

▼ operational or logistical access;

▼ geographic access;

▼ seamless transition between all aspects of the system;

▼ consistent, concise, functionally oriented documentation and outcome data looking at process and clinical items and consumer satisfaction; and

▼ key contact person for any problems or concerns.

Once contracts are awarded to an institution (or in the case of care being delivered outside of a contract), the case manager is the watchdog for the managed care companies. Admission directors, medical directors, program managers, and clinical staff will find themselves negotiating, discussing, and justifying their services to the case manager. Case managers are requiring frequent progress reports for their patients and in many situations will authorize only a small number of sessions at a time. Continuation of clinical services will depend on the actual progress of the patient toward the goals the case manager believes are appropriate.

Many health care organizations have begun to employ internal case managers (sometimes known as care coordinators or like titles) to deal directly with the external case managers. These internal case managers act as liaisons between the clinical staff and the external case managers; they ensure that all appropriate documentation and communication occurs in a timely manner. They also handle the reauthorization process for continuation of any clinical services.

CHANGES IN FACILITY-BASED CLINICAL PRACTICE

The delivery of OT services has changed in many ways:

▼ The length of stay for inpatients has shortened significantly.

- Managed care case managers—not the physician or the treating clinician—are deciding how much of what specific service will be given to the patient.

- Outpatient delivery of service is much more prevalent.

- Goals that were previously attained while a rehab patient was an inpatient are now attained in the OP setting.

- The ratio of professional staff to nonprofessional staff is changing.

- There is much higher use of the less expensive (COTA) or OT aide in OT departments, and there is broad use of the cross-trained, "multiskilled" aide.

- Therapists are expected to treat more than one person at a time—concurrent treatments.

- Many departments are pairing (OTRs) with OT aides as a treatment team to treat two or three patients at once.

These changes have caused new models of delivery of care to be developed in many institutions. There are at least five basic steps in designing new models for care delivery:

Step I: Identify the present model for delivery of clinical service (e.g., each patient is seen one on one for one to two hours of occupational therapy per day; productivity standards are five to six treatment hours per day per therapist).

Step II: Determine the cost of delivering one hour of clinical service.

Cost Analysis

- cost of individual staff salary + benefits

- nonlabor directs within departments (operational budget *minus* salaries; e.g., office supplies, educational expenses, patient treatment supplies, computer supplies)

- productive versus nonproductive factor for the department

- institutional indirects (e.g., cost of operation/administration, institutional debt, housekeeping, accounting department)

Step III: Identify alternate (less expensive) models for delivery of care (see Step IV for examples).

Step IV: Calculate the expected revenue generation for each model and compare that against expected reimbursement per visit from managed care contracts.

- ▼ 1 OTR and 1 aide seeing 3 patients per hour generates 3 x $85 = $255 if 1 hour is charged at $85 per patient.

- ▼ Managed care company is reimbursing at $70 per hour.

- ▼ The *cost* of 1 OTR and 1 aide for 1 hour = $88.

Therefore, the profit on 1 hour, *if* 3 patients are seen, is $122. You need *more* volume per hour to make money from managed care reimbursement. Knowing your *cost* is more important than your *charge*.

Step V: Identify any related factors (e.g., documentation, education, space).

Examples of Alternate Service Delivery Models

* 1 OTR teamed with 1 OT aide seeing 3 patients in session

* 1 OTR teamed with 1 COTA treating a larger caseload than either could carry alone

* 1 COTA teamed with 1 OT aide for group sessions

* Design of programs that use group treatment rather than all individual sessions

70

This transformed practice environment has necessitated a major shift in mind-set for occupational therapy practitioners. With the increases in nonprofessional staff, OTRs have had to become more proficient as supervisors and case managers. The OTR role will increasingly become one of evaluator, communicator, educator, and trainer. The COTA or OT aide will provide the bulk of the hands-on care. The OTR has had to become more skillful in managing the care provided to his or her patients by another individual. Now more than ever, OTRs need to recognize how often professional intervention or reassessment is needed for their patients.

Very stringent competencies have to be developed in each department for the aides now being used more frequently. Detailed orientations and comprehensive education/training sessions have to be provided for the aides to ensure sound performance. Clear, definitive boundaries and role delineation are needed to guarantee quality care by skilled individuals, each doing what they have been trained to do.

Due to the increased productivity expectations related to the new delivery of care models, occupational therapy practitioners are busier. The systems of the institution must support the occupational therapy practitioner for this to be successful. The documentation needs to be streamlined and made as efficient and user friendly as possible. There needs to be adequate space for the increased number of patients seen at the same time. Patients also need to be prepared for the way in which their care will be delivered. Being clear about what to expect during a treatment session will prevent customer dissatisfaction.

Documentation has been mentioned from the practitioner's point of view. Additionally, case managers have very specific expectations for the type of documentation they want. To meet the needs of a managed care environment, documentation must

- ▼ be timely;

- ▼ be integrated for multiple services;

- ▼ be functionally oriented (it must address very specific functional goal attainment; there should be no reductionistic jargon [e.g., "ambulation has increased"; instead, "patient can ambulate from bed to bathroom independently"];

- ▼ address specific goal attainment and functional outcomes;

- ▼ give a specific plan and time line for goal attainment; and

- ▼ give a very accurate "snapshot" of the patient.

Critical paths or Care Maps™ have become an essential type of documentation in this new era. They provide very specific guideposts for clinical care and help ensure consistency per diagnostic group. The pathways/maps give the opportunity to record variances from the expected course of treatment. They also furnish managed care companies very clear information on the product they are considering purchasing and what can be expected in a predetermined length of time.

Another important difference in the delivery of clinical services is the shift in where or on what part of the continuum services are delivered. Case managers are looking for a lower cost alternative to traditional inpatient care. Some examples include

- ▼ subacute or skilled nursing facilities

- ▼ subacute beds within existing facility structures (e.g., acute care hospitals, rehabilitation facilities, skilled nursing facilities)

- ▼ day treatment programs

- ▼ out patient services

- ▼ home care

If an inpatient admission is authorized, the case manager may approve only certain clinical services. Gone are the days when all patients received all services available. Varying treatment models to fit the type of reimbursement is a challenge for today's practitioner.

To be successful, all patients cannot be treated using the same model. The patient's insurance will influence what and how services are delivered to patients.

Again, the driving force here is cost; only those services viewed as essential to that specific patient by the case manager will be authorized. We have entered the era of differing levels of care within the same clinical program with decisions not based on traditional criteria. However, in learning to function in this new era, quality, individual outcomes, and consumer satisfaction must be kept in the equation.

THE HOME CARE PERSPECTIVE

Organizational Changes

As with other settings, home health is focusing on cost reduction to stay competitive in this changing environment. This is being done by flattening the organization chart, monitoring productivity, and computerizing each home visitor. The industry itself has been broadening its scope through an increase in service offerings as with intravenous therapy and respiratory and cardiac specialty services. There may also be a change from the per-visit to the by-unit method of billing.

More home health agencies are moving toward the for-profit entity and away from the freestanding, not-for-profit agencies of the past. Skilled nursing facilities are beginning to develop their own home health agencies and will extend their staff from the long term care arena into the home. Because of the proliferation of skilled nursing facilities throughout the country, this will mean more rural consumers will receive home health services at a minimal travel expense to the agency.

Changes in Clinical Practice

Changes in delivery of service include the following:

▼ The frequency and duration of patient treatment will be increasingly abbreviated.

▼ Patients and caretakers will assume more responsibility for advocating for the amount of care they need. This they must do while they are ill.

▼ Patients and caretakers will assume greater amounts of more complex care.

▼ The ratio of professional to nonprofessional staff will increase with COTAs on the high end of the formula and OTRs assuming more of a consultative role.

▼ There is also concern that inadequately skilled personnel may cover services in order to maximize visits (i.e., the inappropriate use of home health aides in ADLs).

- ▼ Parts of assessments that contain nonskilled questions may be asked of the patient or caretaker by a secretary by telephone prior to the therapist's visit.

- ▼ Some agencies may work from a pre-operative basis—evaluating the patient's post-operative needs.

- ▼ Computerization and voice mail may decrease treatment team effectiveness by eliminating dialogue and the transmission of facts important to treatment.

- ▼ The treating therapists will be required to identify risk to the payer via communications with the internal and external case managers—education will be accomplished through exceptional documentation of treatment plan specifics and the expected outcome if the treatment is not performed.

- ▼ Therapists will need to recognize that patients purchase insurance with specific limits and that a patient may have the option to self-pay for further needed treatment (i.e., 100 visits per calendar year for all home health disciplines—this is easily used in the first 60 days with a CVA patient). This must be communicated tactfully to the patient.

- ▼ The therapist will need to relate to the patients their responsibility in treatment and for continuing their programs after discharge.

- ▼ It is expected that the OT management in home health will be relieved of any administrative duties and, therefore, student programs will be negotiated from the larger health system, as will research efforts.

- ▼ The benefit of home health agencies' becoming part of larger health systems will be improvement in the continuity of patient care; that is, if the patient is followed by the same therapist. Another benefit will be to the system itself by increasing cost-effectiveness through decreasing the duplication of services.

- ▼ Homebound status may be more loosely applied in helping provide the patient a bridge back into the community. This will be applied on a case-by-case basis and is likely to occur first in the mental health arena.

It is most important that home health practitioners know that the most powerful tools in helping their patients obtain the visits needed in the managed care environment is the identification of risk to the payer, the development of a relationship with the internal and external case managers, and their notification when goals are met under the prescribed duration.

THE MENTAL HEALTH PERSPECTIVE

Organizational Changes

The primary method for addressing the cost of behavioral health care services has been the provision of fewer treatment services and/or alternative, less costly services. For example, individuals are being diverted from costly inpatient stays in acute care hospital units to less costly treatment settings: intermediate care facilities that provide 24-hour supervision, partial hospitalization programs, outpatient treatment, or home health treatment.

> ...health care systems need to increase their membership to spread the risk.

In addition to decreasing staff to decrease hospital costs, some institutions are contracting for services outside the institution; in essence, they are managing competition of providers. This may present an opportunity for occupational therapists to provide an expanded range of services that combines certain services other mental health professionals have traditionally provided (e.g., resource management) with more traditional occupational therapy intervention, providing both at less cost.

In addition to increasing the volume of services provided, health care systems need to increase their membership to spread the risk. Thus, costs for individuals with greater need for services can be offset by those with lesser needs. In a public system of statewide services, enrollment is recommended at 300,000 or more. Several additional criteria are important to managed behavioral health care systems:

▼ Providers' services are member/client driven and are focused on consumer satisfaction.

▼ Providers' services are culturally significant.

▼ "Wraparound" concept—services are provided to adults and children where needed (e.g., client's home, jail, school) and include nontraditional services (e.g, a homeless person with serious mental illness is helped to locate and move into a residence).

▼ Services may be provided that seem outside the traditional definition of "medical necessity," but that are needed to maintain the individual's mental stability and functional performance and to avoid using more costly services.

▼ Clients/members have 24-hour access to services; this provides a "safety net" and prevents the use of more costly services; for example, inpatient hospitalization of a disoriented client who arrives at the emergency room at 2:00 A.M. (In one county, all members of a certain managed care service are so identified in county-wide database, and emergency room personnel must contact the provider prior to admission.)

▼ A single fixed point of responsibility is identified for each client/member; it may be an individual or a team.

Case management of services for people with serious mental disorders is often provided by a team, rather than an individual. The team also provides direct services to the individual. In other instances, an individual within the behavioral health care organization determines the need for services and refers the client/member to appropriate service providers in his or her community.

Changes in Clinical Practice

In mental health practice, occupational therapists are increasing their contact and use of the patient's family and significant others. These individuals are now viewed as treatment extenders, in contrast to the past, when the family was often excluded from services and the patient's treatment plan. Because inpatient stays are significantly shortened (from weeks or months to days), occupational therapy services in inpatient settings are changing dramatically. Hospitals are choosing to use their mental health occupational therapists in a variety of ways.

Therapists may be involved most in evaluation to determine the discharge plan rather than treatment. Some therapists are providing service in partial hospital programs or in the patient's home; some therapists with mental health expertise are being used to consult for patients with diagnoses of physical illnesses or injuries. Therapists may be designing and overseeing a patient activity program for people with mental illness diagnoses housed in an acute or intermediate care facility or in group living situations.

Outpatient programs for people with mental disorders are also changing. Traditional day treatment services, for example, may be provided for only half rather than a full day, or for fewer days of the week. Therapeutic efforts may be more strongly directed to community integration or home activities during those times when a day activity program is not provided.

It should be noted that in numerous situations, occupational therapy practitioners may be *less* expensive staff than other mental health personnel, such as a psychiatrist or psychologist. This represents another opportunity for occupational therapists in the changing mental health practice environment. Previously, billing was usually for certain specific services, (e.g., psychotherapy, psychological testing, medication management, or rehabilitation). Payment for such services was limited to certain professionals who were designated as appropriate providers of such services.

This concept itself is being challenged in the treatment of mental disorders on many fronts. In a public managed care system in southern California, only two rates for billing exist. The first is for medication prescription/management; the second is for all other services. *All* providers bill this way—including consumer providers, occupational therapists, noncertified psychiatric workers, and psychiatrists.

Examples of Alternative Service Delivery Models

Occupational therapy practitioners working in behavioral health systems often work as a member of a multidisciplinary team, rather than with other occupational therapy staff. A therapist may direct a multidisciplinary team (which does not necessarily contain another OTR or COTA). A single OTR or COTA is often the only occupational therapy practitioner in a facility or system. The OT practitioner may have a consultative or directive role, rather than a role of direct service provision.

With regard to the competencies of nonlicensed providers or aides providing service for people with mental disorders, several issues need to be considered. First, orientation and ongoing training should reflect the perspective of the payer of the services. Competency training may need to occur on the job to lessen costs. Second, competencies need to be defined at the lowest level and then upward along a continuum. Mental health consumers are hired and used as providers in some settings. Some states have defined scope of practice in their laws that included consumers as providers of mental health services and as such are not necessarily tied to licensure. ▼

76

Reimbursement Issues in Managed Care Delivery Systems

OVERVIEW

Payment methods for services under managed care delivery "systems" are more complex than what have generally been established for traditional, indemnity-type, health plans. One reason is that the concept of service under managed care can have a broader range of meanings. More important, the payment structure of a managed care organization (MCO) is often linked to the individual "managed care" goals of that organization.

A simple definition for the primary objective of all managed care plans is to contain health care costs through various means while ensuring high quality care. Central to the managed care concept are financial incentives and risk for employers, providers, and consumers.

Historically in health care, quality was often associated with quantity and the financial risk lay with the insurer and the employer, with little responsibility on the part of the provider or consumer. Managed care has changed these relationships to the degree that the dollar amount of payment for a service is only one part of the means to arrive at the overall goal of containing costs. The "systems" of providing health care are of paramount importance, and reimbursement can be understood only in relationship to the components of those systems.

It helps first to examine some of the various types of managed care organizations, specifically health maintenance organizations (HMOs) and preferred provider organizations (PPOs), and then to look at how the differences in structure affect patient access to care, provider, and employer incentives. A single insurance company may be an MCO or offer a range of different health plan products with different coverage rules and payment structures, some or all of which may include a managed care approach. Variations in MCOs are usually defined by the relationship between the health plan and its affiliated physicians (primarily those in the gatekeeper roles).

HEALTH MAINTENANCE ORGANIZATIONS

Although HMOs vary in organizational structure, they contain some of the same attributes. In exchange for a prepaid premium, HMO members receive a comprehensive group of health care services. Services are usually provided by a predetermined group of providers either as employees of or under contract to the HMO, and the scope and amount of services received by a member are controlled through a primary care provider (PCP), usually a physician.

The four most common HMO structures are the group model, the staff model, the network model, and the independent practice association (IPA) model. Except for the staff model, physician (i.e., PCP) payment is often on a capitated, rather than a fee-for-service basis.

Staff model	An HMO employs and pays salaries to physicians to provide care.
Group model	An HMO contracts with one independent practice group under an exclusive contract.
Network model	An HMO contracts with two or more physician groups.
IPA model	An HMO contracts with solo physicians and/or group practices to provide care.

PREFERRED PROVIDER ORGANIZATIONS

A preferred provider organization arranges for health care services to be delivered by a network of "preferred" providers who are subject to the PPO's managed care controls, such as use of case management and utilization review. PPOs provide a large referral base for preferred, or "in-plan," providers and generally pay based on a discounted fee-for-service method. Although members have the option of receiving care from "out-of-network" providers, there are significant financial disincentives in the form of benefit restrictions and co-payments for doing so.

POINT OF SERVICE

A point-of-service plan, which is sometimes referred to as a *mixed-model plan*, provides additional flexibility by allowing the consumer to choose to follow the HMO managed care rules (e.g., PCP referrals, use of network providers) or choose to go outside the network *at the time of service* rather than being locked into an enrollment decision. However, as in a PPO, there are usually financial disincentives for opting out of the network.

EVOLVING PAYMENT SYSTEMS: CAPITATION AND RISK

Fee for Service—Traditionally, providers have been paid on the basis of some type of rate per unit of service (e.g., procedure code or per diem). This rate may be based on a fee schedule or may be a negotiated rate for a specific treatment or groups of treatments. Generally under fee for service, a practitioner is paid for each code or service billed and has no incentive to limit procedures and tests or to examine lower cost types of treatment. In a fee-for-service system, the insurer assumes primary risk, since under the contractual provisions with the employer/consumer, the insurer must pay for all covered care. For this reason, payers often use cost-saving techniques such as preset service limitations or postpayment utilization reviews to identify overutilization by providers.

    Capitation—In a capitated system, the provider is paid prospectively, usually on a monthly basis, for each member of a specific population (e.g., health plan, Medicaid) regardless of whether any covered health care service is delivered. This prospective rate is termed *per member per month* (PMPM) and is customarily based on the past claims experience of the specific capitated population. Under capitation, the provider has the benefit of a predictable revenue source, but is at greater financial risk, since more service equals less profit. For a provider, the PMPM amount is the most important factor in determining the profitability, or even the feasibility, of a capitated contract.

WHO GETS CAPITATED?

Capitation provisions are primarily found in HMO contracts, since this type of MCO is the most homogeneous in terms of administrative and utilization controls. However, legal affiliations and payment relationships among hospitals, clinics, laboratories, and other types of health care providers are continually evolving, and forms of capitated payment are being used in other types of networks. Capitation rates were developed initially for primary care provider payment. This payment method is more easily (and equitably) calculated for PCPs, who as "gatekeepers" have the most patient interaction and control of services. Additionally, it is easier to project service cost and therefore to set a valid PMPM rate.

    Many HMOs continue to pay specialists—whether physicians, therapists, or other provider types—on a fee-for-service basis. As provider chains and multispecialty organizations continue to grow, it becomes easier to statistically estimate the amount of treatment that a prospectively set PMPM rate should cover without the risk of catastrophic loss to the provider. When physicians, IPAs, specialty rehabilitation groups, and/or hospitals are capitated, therapy services are sometimes subcontracted to another entity that may be paid under a different method.

In addition to the PMPM amount, providers should consider all aspects of a contract in evaluating the viability of a capitation arrangement. Some of these factors follow:

Number of members in the capitated population	The greater the number, the higher the overall prospectively paid monthly rate from that plan will be.
Member profile	Risk (i.e., use of services) is statistically determined by age, sex, and health care factors relative to the type of service provided.
Specific details of the plan that affect the members' access to and incentives to use services	Benefit package, member deductibles and co-payment amounts, referral requirements (e.g., requirements that care is referred by a PCP) or a high co-payment for therapy will reduce demand for services. For example, a provider may require a higher capitation rate to offset a low co-pay.
Number of other similar providers in the network	Generally, if there are few providers offering similar services, the PMPM rate must be high enough to cover the cost of an expected large number of referrals.

RISK-SHARING ARRANGEMENTS UNDER CAPITATION

The concept of "risk sharing" and the construction of "risk pools" are critical issues for provider decisions on whether to join capitated networks. However, risk adjustments can also exist in other noncapitated contractual arrangements. A risk pool of dollars is created from a designated amount of money withheld from provider payments throughout the year and used to meet specified expenses of the pool.

Based on a predefined "reward" formula, unused funds in the pool are distributed at the end of the year to those providers who meet the targeted use and/or cost goals. The design of the pool (e.g., specialties of providers, number per pool) and how it is used during the year determine the risk (e.g., whether there is any money in the pool by the end of the year). There is an infinite number of arrangements and formulas that can be created under the guise of "risk sharing," and providers should always understand the details of each contract to which they commit.

MANAGED CARE IS NOT JUST CAPITATION

As stated, payment rates and contract pricing are just one part of a managed care strategy. Most insurers are infusing managed care principles into their more "traditional" indemnity products in addition to HMO and PPO type plans. Following are some of the management techniques commonly used to control costs and quality.

▼ Case management—Especially for long-term and/or high cost cases, insurers use case managers, often employed outside the plan, to oversee and designate which group of services will yield the best outcome. Often, this decision-making power allows a case manager to approve treatments that may not be normally covered by a plan. Some insurers use the terms *case management* and *managed care* synonymously.

▼ Precertification or preauthorization—The requirement that specific tests, surgical procedures, or categories of services (e.g., mental health) be authorized before allowed gives the insurer the opportunity to deny "unnecessary" treatment and/or substitute lower cost services.

▼ Mandatory second opinion before approval of any or specific types of surgical procedures.

▼ Use of a third-party administrator—This is a private company that specializes in management of various administrative (e.g., claims) and managed care (e.g., utilization review) functions of a plan or an employer (if self-insured).

MANAGED CARE IN PUBLICLY FUNDED PROGRAMS

Most publicly funded insurance programs have incorporated managed care techniques in an effort to hold down rising health care costs. A managed care philosophy is now evident in the administration of Medicare, Medicaid, Civilian Health and Medical Program of the Uniformed Services, and many state-based workers' compensation programs.

MEDICARE MANAGED CARE

When the Medicare program was created in 1965, it covered most people 65 years of age and older. In 1973, new legislation extended coverage to people entitled to disability benefits for 24 months or longer, people with end-stage renal disease (ESRD) requiring dialysis or kidney transplant, and certain noncovered beneficiaries who decide to purchase Medicare coverage on their own.

Although about 95 percent of Medicare beneficiaries in 1994 were enrolled in a traditional Medicare plan (i.e., on a fee-for-service indemnity basis), a growing number of Medicare beneficiaries are expected to join managed care plans in the future. Medicare beneficiaries enrolled in Parts A and B, or in Part B only, may elect to join managed care plans that have been certified and awarded a contract by the U.S. Health Care Financing Administration (HCFA), which administers the Medicare program. Under this arrangement, HCFA pays most HMOs a monthly capitated (per enrolled beneficiary) amount on behalf of the beneficiary for all Medicare covered services except hospice care (which managed care plans are not mandated to cover).

A smaller number of managed care plans, including preferred provider organizations, have been awarded contracts by HCFA but are paid under a fee-for-service, reasonable-cost methodology. Each plan must be able to deliver with "reasonable promptness" all medically necessary services that Medicare beneficiaries are entitled to receive and that are available to Medicare beneficiaries living in the same geographic area but who are not enrolled in a managed care plan. When medically necessary, services must be continuously available and accessible.

Most managed care plans typically cover all preventive, acute, and subacute health services on a prepaid basis. Although specific cost-sharing levels will vary according to policies established by each plan, the beneficiary is often required to pay a supplemental premium for "medigap" coverage of Medicare deductibles, Medicare coinsurance, or services not covered by Medicare. The standard Medicare Part B premium is always required.

Through the optional Medicare Select program, available in some states, beneficiaries can purchase supplemental medigap policies through managed care plans that are less expensive than medigap plans offered under traditional indemnity insurance. In return, these beneficiaries must obtain health care services from providers affiliated with the Medicare select plan's provider network. Health care practitioners are either salaried or paid by managed care plans under capitated or discounted fee-for-service rates.

MEDICARE BENEFICIARIES EXPERIENCES WITH MANAGED CARE PLANS

In a 1993 U.S. Office of the Inspector General survey, disabled or ESRD beneficiaries who disenrolled from a Medicare HMO reported access to care problems more frequently than aged beneficiaries, and 66 percent of disabled/ESRD enrollees surveyed wanted to leave their HMOs. However, a majority of all beneficiaries surveyed (including both the aged and disabled/ESRD populations) joined another HMO after disenrollment.

MEDICARE POINT-OF-SERVICE OPTION

HCFA recently announced a new Medicare point-of-service insurance option that will permit HMO beneficiaries to seek care outside the HMO's provider network, typically at higher cost-sharing levels than in-network care. HCFA does not mandate that selected services or providers be made available out of network. Instead, each plan specifies the providers and services that can be accessed outside of the HMO provider network.

MEDICAID MANAGED CARE

Medicaid is a health care entitlement program serving primarily low-income families and their children and aged, blind, and disabled low-income people. The program is financed and administered jointly by each state and the federal government. Under federal law, each state must deliver certain health services to people meeting federal poverty level standards and individuals eligible for the Aid to Families with Dependent Children (AFDC) and Supplemental Security Income (SSI) programs. Each state is also allowed to cover additional populations or services not required by the federal government, and OT is considered a separate optional Medicaid service. The types of individuals covered and the extent of OT coverage, therefore, vary widely depending on policies developed by each state.

83

Currently, state governments may apply to the federal government for a waiver that will allow Medicaid beneficiaries to enroll in managed care plans. Once a state waiver is approved by the federal government, managed care plans are awarded contracts by the state to deliver services, using both federal and state approval criteria. A Section 1915(b) (of the U.S. Social Security Act) federal waiver allows a state to restrict a beneficiary's choice of provider and is often limited to selected geographic regions within a state. A Section 1115 waiver is a more extensive research and demonstration project that is usually granted for a five-year period. Under Section 1115, states are allowed to test major changes in the way Medicaid services are delivered. Under most Section 1115 waivers, the existing benefits packages, including OT benefits, that were available before the waiver was approved continue to be made available through a managed care plan contractor. However, the risk of having services limited is increased when case management, coverage decisions, and utilization review authority are transferred from the state government to a managed care plan.

Most state waivers have focused enrollment in managed care plans on the AFDC population, which primarily comprises women and children with routine care needs, rather than the SSI population, which is primarily made up of disabled beneficiaries with more expensive chronic care needs. According to a recent major study, "States have been cautious about extending managed care to SSI populations, in part because relatively few managed care

organizations have developed expertise in managing special needs of these populations..."
(Lewin-VHI, 1995). However, the District of Columbia government recently announced a
research demonstration project that will enroll disabled children on Medicaid in managed
care plans on a voluntary basis.

CHAMPUS MANAGED CARE

When military treatment facilities are not needed or are unavailable, the Civilian Health and
Medical Program of the Uniformed Services (CHAMPUS) contracts with private health care
providers for services to active-duty military personnel, military retirees, or dependents of
active-duty military personnel or military retirees.

Under a new TRICARE benefit that was announced in 1995, CHAMPUS beneficiaries will receive services through either an HMO or PPO option, or continue to be covered under conventional CHAMPUS indemnity insurance. To implement the program, the
Department of Defense has awarded TRICARE contracts to private managed care plans
throughout the country. The standard CHAMPUS benefits package will continue to be
available through each TRICARE plan.

WORKERS' COMPENSATION MANAGED CARE

Workers' compensation programs are financed jointly by individual employers or groups
of employers and each state government. Each state develops workers' compensation laws
that determine whether an employer is required to participate, the financial responsibility
of the employer, the benefits provided and workers covered, and the way in which the
insurance is administered. Workers' compensation insurance may be administered through
a private insurance plan under contract with the state or through individual or groups of
employers who administer their own programs (also known as self-insurance).

Due to a rapid rise in workers' compensation costs in the last several years, many states
and employers who self-insure have been contracting with managed care organizations as a
way of lowering costs. In a recent national survey of 250 HMOs, 51 percent reported providing managed care services for patients under a workers' compensation plan. According to
the survey, the primary cost-containment strategies used by HMOs included large case management, utilization review protocols, and return-to-work programs. ▼

REFERENCE

Lewin-VHI, Inc. (1995). *States as payers: Managed care for Medicaid populations.* National
    Institute for Health Care Management.

The Case Manager in Case Management

As health care moves into the 21st century, the increased visibility of case managers is projected. It is important for occupational therapy practitioners to understand the role and function of case managers in order to survive in this changing health care environment of managed care.

The Case Management Society of America (CMSA) defines *case management* as "a collaborative process which assesses, plans, implements, coordinates, monitors and evaluates options and services to meet an individual's health needs through communication and available resources to promote quality cost-effective outcomes."

CMSA describes the case manager as being in the role of health care coordination. CMSA believes that the case manager must have at minimum positive relationship building skills, effective written and verbal communication, and the ability to effect change, perform critical analysis, plan, and promote client/family autonomy. The case manager must also have knowledge of funding resources, services, and clinical standards and outcomes.

This last area is where "lay" case managers have difficulty. They are unsure of those diagnostic procedures that are inappropriate or what a reasonable length of stay might be for a certain injury or diagnosis. With time, many acquire this knowledge. Also, many insurance companies employ or contract with health care providers to consult and review those cases the lay managers identify as difficult. Most of the time these consultants are nurses. The CMSA has established Standards of Practice for Case Management, which are expected to be followed by all certified case managers (CCMs).

Case management is not new. It has existed for many years in the workers' compensation and automobile insurance industries. It has also been a component in established health maintenance organizations. The concept of case management encompasses the entire spectrum of disability claims administration. People have been claiming disability for several decades. To determine whether a claim was appropriate, it was given to an adjustor. Today, that same person may be referred to as the *case manager*. However, this is inappropriate, as we will discuss.

A case management system is designed to provide guidelines for policyholder and claimant relationships, information gathering, file documentation and action, rehabilitation, claim termination, management controls, and other claim-related activities. However, that does not make the individual performing these tasks necessarily a case manager.

Case management evolved to maximize health care expenditures by allocating resources to the most appropriate and effective care. Case management has strong roots in the basic social casework method, which is predicated on assessment of the client and client system, appropriate intervention, and follow-up to ensure continuity and/or closure. Acceptance of case management as a standard in health care is evolving; therefore, medical professionals, employers, and the public at large are likely to interact with case managers.

An understanding of case management can promote more cooperative and productive endeavors and thus better outcomes. It is the outcomes that one uses to determine if the case was managed appropriately or to reflect differences in providers of similar services. Case management differs from managed care in that managed care strategies are designed to accommodate large numbers of people, such as enrollees in a group insurance plan. Case management, on the other hand, applies to a relatively small segment of the population receiving facility-based services. It has been said that 2 percent of the population consumes about 30 percent of all hospital resources in the United States. This group of high-cost users is why medical case management developed.

Actually, there are five basic case management models: medical case management, primary case management, disability case management, social case management, and vocational case management. Although these differ in the types of needs they address and solutions they propose, the approach of case management is similar. Frequently, circumstances change but the basic case management process does not. [In each model, the functions of a case manager are typically to help the patient/client receive the best care and to control the costs.]

There are internal and external case managers. Many health care facilities have identified a person inhouse to serve as the case manager for each patient/client. The in-house or internal case manager is usually a clinical person and frequently a direct service provider to the patient/client (e.g., nurse, social worker, therapist). The external case manager is typically one who is assigned to the case by a payer, such as an insurance company.

Sometimes there is a case manager for the employer, especially when it is large and self-insured. In such cases, the internal case manager acts a liaison between the facility/provider and the external case manager. The internal case manager rarely has influence in the financing of services; he or she is expected to communicate the justification for services the facility/provider is supplying. The external case manager approves and endorses the services. Finances and length of services are two issues the external case manager is expected to "control," while attempting to obtain the most appropriate outcome. Ongoing communication is critical throughout the process.

HOW TO BECOME A CERTIFIED CASE MANAGER

To earn the designation of CCM, an individual must pass the national certification examination. A potential examinee must first show evidence (through documentation) that he or she possesses an acceptable minimum level of basic knowledge of the case management process. The initial certification is valid for five years. The applicant for certification must satisfy specific educational and employment requirements and pass the CCM examination. The examination is based on a body of knowledge that encompasses laws, public regulations, insurance language, and delivery of case management services in the United States.

There are six categories in which an individual must qualify for eligibility to enter the certification process. The certification process excludes individuals who are not health and human services professionals. Certification must be maintained through continuing education opportunities.

For further information on becoming a certified case manager, contact CIRSC/Certified Case Manager, 1835 Rohlwing Road, Suite D, Rolling Meadows, IL 60008; phone (708) 818-0292.

It is the external case manager with whom the occupational therapy practitioner must interact in the workplace. Other types of case managers include the certified rehabilitation counselor or the certified insurance rehabilitation specialist. Again, other external case managers are lay people who have had on-the-job training. Regardless, they are key players and critical individuals in this era of managed care.

OT practitioners need to understand where the particular case manager is "coming from" on any given case, and they must work collaboratively. In this way, case managers will meet their objective of managing the case effectively with an appropriate outcome and the OTs will succeed in assisting the patient/client in attaining his or her functional goals of occupational performance.

CASE MANAGEMENT FROM A MENTAL HEALTH PERSPECTIVE

Although not all providers agree with the present designation, mental health and substance abuse treatment services are now collectively termed *behavioral health care*. Behavioral health care differs from other kinds of medical care in that there are two systems. One is financed through Medicaid and state or county mental health departments and is generally referred to as the *public sector.* The other system is usually referred to as *private* and includes payment from private insurers, individuals paying out of pocket, and Medicare.

Individuals diagnosed with serious mental illness (e.g., schizophrenia, bipolar disorder, or a dual diagnosis of a mental illness and substance abuse and/or mental retardation) are most frequently seen in the public system. Individuals diagnosed with conditions such as depressive disorder, substance abuse (alone), and adjustment disorder are typically treated within the private system. This distinction is important in understanding the role of the case manager, as it is somewhat different in these two systems.

> Public managed care systems vary and often differ widely from state to state.

Public managed care systems vary and often differ widely from state to state. These variations are based on the needs of the payer, purchaser of services, providers, and consumers. However, in the public system, an individual with a serious mental illness who is receiving treatment through a managed care entity most likely has a case manager or case management team that provides both case management and *other needed services.*

Team members evaluate the client's needs on an ongoing basis to determine the most appropriate services. Appropriateness is based on identified outcomes that are based on prevention of need for more costly services, consumer desires for outcomes versus services, and a determination of an adequate— though not always optimum—standard of living. Families and significant others are becoming more involved in this process as they are viewed as treatment extenders to the client within his or her natural environment.

In the private system of care, the case manager does not usually provide treatment services. Rather, he or she has more of a role in service authorization and health care coordination, including some or all of the following: assessment of need, overall treatment plan, monitoring of service delivery, and revision of plan as needed. The level of involvement may vary among behavioral health care plans and may be based on the severity and chronicity of the mental illness. Case management is an important mechanism in these plans to control costs, particularly by diverting admissions to acute care inpatient hospital beds.

The following case is an example of an outcome for mental health services (including occupational therapy services) that exemplifies this concept

> Mr. Jones has a diagnosis of schizoaffective disorder. He began experiencing difficulties recently on his part-time job along with an increase in his psychotic symptoms. He was hospitalized after an attempted suicide in response to a command hallucination. Several problems were identified while he was hospitalized. He lives alone in a single-room hotel and has few friends or activities outside of the two half-days he works at the local soup kitchen. Further, he has difficulty taking his medication correctly and managing his finances.

> Since his symptoms have cleared, he is to be discharged from the hospital. An occupational therapist heads a community treatment team. Mr. Jones will be referred to this team for case management and other needed services. Mr. Jones' goals are to get a part-time job and improve his physical condition. The case management team's goals will be to address his functional problems to prevent rehospitalization for at least six months.

> Establishing a medication regimen, a plan of action for when he begins having suicidal thoughts, and a plan for managing his money will be priorities immediately upon discharge. The team will also enter Mr. Jones into the database used by the emergency rooms of the local public hospitals. The emergency room staff will then know to contact the case management team member on call if and when Mr. Jones comes to the emergency room. Then they will help Mr. Jones begin to engage in regular physical activities and find—and keep—a part-time job.

In this example, the focus of the case management team is to address problems of function rather than merely freedom from symptoms. The result of the team's intervention will then assist in decreasing the costs of care for Mr. Jones over time. In addition, Mr. Jones is assisted in breaking his cycle of repeated hospitalizations resulting in loss of jobs and social contacts. While optimum functioning for Mr. Jones might be full-time employment, this may not necessarily be a goal that his team is pursuing. Rather, the focus is stabilization of his current situation. ▼

Outcomes

INTRODUCTION

The health care world of today is undergoing rapid change: from "do more, get paid more" to "do less, get paid less" (Wilkerson, 1995). As managed care and capitated reimbursement grow, demands are being placed on managers and providers to demonstrate the value and outcomes of their services. Many sectors of the health care industry are turning to outcomes measurement and management and program evaluation as essential strategies and tools for survival and adjustment to this changing climate. These processes offer the potential to provide valuable information to external audiences on the effectiveness and efficiency of care; and internally, they are the core of programmatic quality improvement. As resources continue to dwindle, managers need to know how to allocate those resources to produce the best outcomes.

HISTORICAL PERSPECTIVE

The impetus for outcome information dates back to the 1970s. Health care expenditures were rising, and payers were challenging providers to demonstrate that they were "getting their money's worth." In addition, physicians were faced with demands for unlimited care by patients, new and more expensive technologies were being introduced, and the environment was one of defensive medicine. These factors, coupled with some startling statistics, became a resounding wake-up call. Such figures included

- ▼ Health care costs in the United States are projected to be close to $1.7 trillion by 2000.

- ▼ 60 million people are uninsured or marginally insured.

- ▼ 35 million Americans have ongoing disabilities.

- ▼ 20–30 percent of all medical procedures may not be warranted ($125 billion/year).

- ▼ 20 percent of all health care expenditures are administrative costs.

In the early 1970s, a series of small-area analysis studies was carried out by John Wennenberg, MD, of the Dartmouth Medical School (Wennenberg and Gittlesohn, 1973). Now considered seminal work, Wennenberg was able to demonstrate substantial variability in patterns of medical care within small geographic areas. These variations in levels of health care use were due to physician beliefs, training, practice patterns, hospital beds, number of specialists in a given area versus the health status of the population.

The industry continued to experience widespread variations in the patterns and delivery of health care services; costs of care were spiraling out of control; providers were needing to make resource allocation decisions; and there were growing demands to assess the quality of care. The initial movement was driven by the effort to document value. However, as researchers began to look at cost-effectiveness, they found that by examining the processes by which care was delivered, the quality improved in several situations. Interest grew in integrating cost-effectiveness and quality, with outcomes as the yardstick for both. This, in turn, led to the alphabet soup of *QI*, *QA*, and *QM* programs and activities.

In summary, there was a growing belief that by using improved methods of service delivery (critical pathways, quality improvement, program evaluation) and outcome information, costs could be reduced and quality improved. This movement to measure the effects of care—and thereby prove its value—was given a name when Paul Ellwood, MD, coined the term *outcomes management* in his May 1988 Shattuck Lecture.

OUTCOME EVALUATION

An outcome is the result of a process. It is the status of the patient after care has been provided (i.e., the end result of care). Outcome measurement is the systematic, quantitative observation, at a point in time of outcome indicators. Other definitions include the following:

▼ "Outcome evaluation concentrates on the results of services, programs, treatment or intervention strategies generally following termination of services or during a predetermined follow-up period" (CARF, 1979).

▼ "Outcome evaluation is a systematic procedure for monitoring the effectiveness and efficiency with which results are achieved by persons served as well as customer satisfaction following termination of services" (Forer, 1987).

▼ "Outcomes Management is the use of information and knowledge gained from outcome monitoring to achieve optimal patient outcomes through improved clinical decision-making and service delivery" (Davies et al., 1994).

▼ "An occupational therapy outcome is the functional consequence for the patient of the therapeutic action implemented by an occupational therapist" (Rogers and Holm, 1994).

PURPOSES OF OUTCOME EVALUATION

The following is reprinted from the AOTA publication, *A Resource Guide on Outcome Management and Program Evaluation for Occupational Therapy Practitioners* (Forer, 1996).

The main reasons for conducting outcome evaluation are to (1) improve client benefits (effectiveness), (2) improve efficiency (resource management), and (3) justify, maintain, or expand funding and general community support. An occupational therapy outcome is the functional consequence for the patient of the therapeutic interventions rendered by an occupational therapy practitioner. However, the temptation of many practitioners is to use refined clinical measures such as range of motion (ROM), muscle strength as measured by a dynamometer, endurance, lifting and reaching capacity rather than measuring the actual functional outcome (i.e., independence in activities of daily living [ADLs], return to work or former lifestyle, quality of life, and general health perception). Although increased ROM, muscle strength and endurance, sensory and motor function, and cognitive and psychosocial function are all important, the key question is what is the patient able to do (perform) as a result of these increased skills. If an increase of 10 percent in ROM does not appear to make any difference in a patient's ability to dress or feed himself or herself, then the intervention may not be perceived as cost-effective. Care should be taken in identifying the expected outcomes and measures for occupational therapy.

Definitions of Impairment, Disability, and Handicap

Unfortunately, the term *function* has many connotations. It may refer to an organ or system of the body, as in neuromuscular function; a task function, as in dressing; or the ability to function in a role that is socially expected, such as worker or homemaker. The World Health Organization (WHO, 1980) model of disablement and definitions of *impairment*, *disability*, and *handicap* provide a conceptual framework for evaluating outcomes and have become widely accepted by rehabilitation professionals and researchers.

Impairment refers to "any loss or abnormality of psychological, physiological or anatomical structure or function." Examples of impairment would include the Impairment Groups from the Uniform Data System for Medical Rehabilitation (UDSMR, 1993), nature and etiology of impairment, Frankel classification for spinal cord injury (American Spinal Injury Association, 1982), ROM, muscle tone, and strength.

Disability refers to "any restriction or lack (resulting from an impairment) of ability to perform an activity in the manner or within the range considered normal for a human being." Disability refers to dysfunction of task performance. Examples include measures of severity of disability or burden of care, such as the Functional Independence Measure, (UDS$_{MR}$, 1993), ADLs, instrumental activities of daily living, mobility, communication, and cognitive and psychosocial adjustment. Most of these measures are based on observed performance and not an assessment of capacity or capability.

Handicap refers to "a disadvantage for a given individual, resulting from an impairment or disability, that limits or prevents the fulfillment of a role that is normal for their age, gender and culture." The WHO definition of handicap includes six areas of role function: orientation, physical independence, mobility, occupation, social integration, and economic self-sufficiency. Handicap is basically the social disadvantage of the impairment and resulting disability. Handicap measures might include work and productive activities, home management, educational and vocational activities, play and leisure, quality of life, and perception of wellness.

A variety of different impairment, disability, and handicap outcome measures may be selected for each occupational therapy practice setting. Most of the postacute, outpatient, work-hardening, home health, and mental health program objectives tend to focus more on the handicap issues, while the acute care, acute rehabilitation, and subacute program objectives tend to focus more on the impairment and disability issues.

Uniform Terminology for Occupational Therapy—The American Occupational Therapy Association has published its third edition of the *Uniform Terminology for Occupational Therapy* (1994). According to this document, *occupational therapy* is the use of purposeful activity or intervention to promote health and achieve functional outcomes. "Achieving functional outcomes" means to develop, improve, or restore the highest possible level of independence of any individual who is limited by a physical injury or illness, a dysfunctional condition, a cognitive impairment, a psychological dysfunction, a mental illness, a developmental or learning disability, or an adverse environmental condition. Occupational therapy focuses on *performance areas, performance components,* and *performance contexts.*

Performance areas are broad categories of *human activity* that are typically part of daily life and include activities of daily living, work and productive activities, and play or leisure activities.

Performance components are fundamental *human abilities* that—to varying degrees and different combinations—are required for successful engagement in performance areas. These components are sensorimotor, cognitive, psychosocial, and psychological.

Performance Contexts are *situations or factors that influence* an individual's engagement in desired and/or performance areas. They may be temporal aspects (chronological, developmental, life cycle, and disability status) and environmental aspects (physical, social, and cultural).

Although function in *performance areas* is the ultimate objective of occupational therapy, function must be evaluated in light of the *performance components* and *performance contexts* that may have a direct impact on the outcomes in the performance areas. For example, a worker who is disabled from a work-related injury may have the potential for returning to work and productive activities. However, to accomplish this, the individual must first develop the strength, endurance, soft tissue integrity, time management, and physical features of the performance contexts. It may be necessary to redesign the work tasks, adjust the workload capacity, or provide vocational retraining or supported employment to enable the individual to return to work.

Emerging Emphasis on Outcomes and Cost-Effectiveness—Until fairly recently, the health care industry and occupational therapy practitioners have focused their attention more on the process of care, timeliness, and appropriateness of treatment. It has only been in the last 7 to 10 years that providers have begun to look more at outcomes. Third-party payers, particularly managed care and workers' compensation carriers, have become increasingly concerned with long-term outcomes, total case costs, and future health care usage. Although a number of outcome measures have been developed for some practice settings, there is still a dearth of outcome measures across the continuum of care. There is no industry consensus over which tools to use or how to use them. In fact, it may be a very unrealistic expectation to choose one outcome measure (gold standard) that is appropriate for all levels of care and practice settings. One thing is clear, however; providers must begin to evaluate the outcomes of their programs and services and to use this information to improve the quality, outcomes, cost effectiveness, and customer satisfaction. The goal of rehabilitation efforts has shifted from *maximize functional recovery and independence* to *optimize functional recovery*, transitioning a patient as soon as possible and when it is safe to do so to the least costly setting, thereby maximizing cost-effectiveness. Under a capitated health care system, providers will be forced to do just that.

USES OF OUTCOME EVALUATION

Outcome data can be used for a variety of purposes. Briefly, they include

- ▼ quality assessment and program modification
- ▼ clinical care and data for research studies
- ▼ planning for future program development
- ▼ marketing; and
- ▼ contract negotiations with managed care companies

CONSIDERATIONS IN CHOOSING/DEVELOPING AN OUTCOME SYSTEM

There are clearly many benefits to the provider and facility for including outcome assessment as a routine part of clinical practice and operations. In addition to the information already outlined, an article entitled "Measure for Measure" (Munro, 1994) presented 10 practical steps to consider when creating and managing outcome systems:

(1) Track information that your managed care companies, payers, and patients and other consumers want to see.

(2) Uses existing resources and professional experts. Don't reinvent the wheel. Build on what others are doing.

(3) Keep it simple. Concentrate on data needed to improve operations and satisfy customers.

(4) Consider uses a national database as part of your overall system. It is important to know how one compares to other providers in a particular region or nationally in terms of case mix, outcome, and resource use.

(5) Collect information on functional outcomes, costs, and patient satisfaction.

(6) Communicate findings with clinical staff and external audiences.

(7) Use your system to complement quality improvement activities.

(8) Consider associated costs (hardware, software, and training), if selecting an automated collection system.

(9) Make training an ongoing process and include all personnel.

(10) Include items that set your program apart from others.

Several years ago, a handout was put together on outcomes and OT practice. It included some relevant predictions for the future. Interestingly, many of these are already taking place. For example

(1) Community-based practices will collect and use outcome data to improve patient care, market their services, and negotiate managed care contracts.

(2) Employers will demand and use outcomes analysis information to select health insurance plans for their employees.

(3) Patients will demand more participation in the clinical decision-making process and will expect better information about the results of health care interventions.

(4) A whole new industry will develop consisting of organizations that specialize in the capture and analysis of outcomes data (Zabludoff, 1993).

A closing quote from Paul Ellwood, MD, clearly summarizes the priority and focus on outcomes: "Rehabilitation will be required to prove its value, as will all other types of health care services. Outcomes management will be the means used to measure the quality of health care provided by an organization.... As health care providers, all of us must demonstrate that what we do is really worthwhile, and we must provide the data on our results that allow such a determination of value" (1988). ▼

REFERENCES

American Occupational Therapy Association. (1994). Uniform terminology for occupational therapy—third edition. *American Journal of Occupational Therapy, 48*(11), 1047–1059.

American Spinal Injury Association. (1982). *Standard for neurological classification of SCI patients.* Chicago, IL: ASIA.

Commission on Accreditation of Rehabilitation Facilities. (1979). *Program evaluation in inpatient medical rehabilitation facilities.* Tucson, AZ: CARF.

Commission on Accreditation of Rehabilitation Facilities. (1995). *1995 standards for medical rehabilitation.* Tucson, AZ: CARF.

Davies, A. R., Doyle, M., Lansky, D., Rutt, W., Stevic, M. O., & Doyle, J. B. (1994). Outcomes assessment in clinical settings. *Journal of Quality Improvement 20*(1), 6–16.

Ellwood, P. (1988). Outcomes management: A technology of patient experience. *New England Journal of Medicine, 318,* 1459.

Fisher, A.G. (1992). Functional measures, part 1: What is function, what should we measure, and how should we measure it? *American Journal of Occupational Therapy, 42*(2), 183–185.

Fisher, A. G., & Short-DeGraff, M. (1993). Improving functional assessment in occupational therapy: Recommendations and philosophy for change. *American Journal of Occupational Therapy, 47*(3), 199–201.

Forer, S. (1987). Outcome analysis for program service management. In M. J. Fuhrer (Ed.), *Rehabilitation outcomes: Analysis and measurement* (pp. 115–136). Baltimore, MD: Paul H. Brookes.

Forer, S. (1996), *Outcome management and program evaluation made easy: A toolkit for occupational therapy practitioners.* Bethesda, MD: American Occupational Therapy Association.

MacDonell, C. (1994). Program evaluation: A management tool for you. *Administration and Management Special Interest Section Newsletter, 10*(2), 2–4.

Munro, D. (1994). Measure for measure. *Rehabilitation Today,* March, 10–19.

Rogers, J. C., & Holm, M. B. (1994). Accepting the challenge of outcome research: Examining the effectiveness of occupational therapy practice. *American Journal of Occupational Therapy, 48*(10), 871–876.

Uniform Data System for Medical Rehabilitation. (1993). *A Guide for the Uniform Data Set for Medical Rehabilitation (Adult FIM), version 4.0.* Buffalo, NY: State University of New York—Buffalo and the Center for Functional Assessment Research.

Wennenberg, J., & Gittelsohn, A. (1973). Small area variations in health care delivery. *Science, 182,* 1102–1108.

Wilkerson, D. L. (1995). Developing outcomes management tools. *Rehabilitation Management,* December–January, 114-117, 129.

World Health Organization. (1980). *International classification of impairments, disabilities, and handicaps* (pp. 21, 45, 47, 181, 183). Geneva: WHO.

Zabludoff, J. (1993). Rehabilitation, outcomes management, and healthcare reform: A conversation with Paul Ellwood, MD, *Rehab Management,* June–July, 30–34.

Managed Care and Ethics

Managed care is an approach to health care delivery that provides for coordination of care as well as monitoring cost and quality control. There are many models of alternative delivery systems. The alternative delivery systems include but are not limited to health maintenance organizations, provider service networks, managed care organizations, and independent practice associations. Occupational therapy practitioners are working in all of these environments. As health care consumers, we are receiving our care through such entities.

What are the ethical conflicts that many experience? The conflicts for the occupational therapy practitioner are the same as those for physicians and other health care providers. How do we contain cost? How do we provide quality care? How do we take into account patient preference? Each of these questions can be simple or complex as in the managed care environment all questions seem to have a monetary component and a patient care component.

However, to answer these questions, occupational therapy practitioners need to understand that health care provided in today's world is provided as a commodity. It is neither unethical nor illegal to look at medicine, and by substitution occupational therapy, as a business. It is neither unethical nor illegal to make a profit from one's expertise. Managed care organizations have a fiduciary duty to the stockholders to maximize profits.

The conflict that comes up most often with occupational therapy practitioners is based on divided loyalty. The divided loyalty is between personal values (quality of care) and institutional values (cost containment). Personal values emphasize the *Core Values and Attitudes of Occupational Therapy Practice* (AOTA, 1993). Truthfulness, promise keeping, and the ethical principle of beneficence (doing what is best for the recipient of service) are in conflict with the institutional values of retreating from provision of more care as defined by the recipient of service to less intensive care provided in a proscribed manner by a third-party payer and/or utilization review organizations.

To ameliorate some of the values conflict, occupational therapy practitioners should look to the *Occupational Therapy Code of Ethics* (AOTA, 1994) as an action guide. The *Code of Ethics* states that the recipient of service should be allowed to be an autonomous decision maker. To do this, one has to have the relevant facts. Occupational therapy practitioners should learn as much as possible about the institutional rules and regulations that are governing the provision of care as well as the goals and aspirations of the patient. Knowledge of these two components that guide your practice should aid in the alleviation of a values conflict. Also, knowledge of specific business practices and how the institutional values mesh with your personal values will aid in alleviating ethical conflicts.

The recipient of service does have something to add to the managed care equation. It must be remembered by all that the recipient of service not only receives the service but pays for the services. If as occupational therapy practitioners we provide something that is seen only as ancillary and not as quality, the word will go out that occupational therapy is not a value for the money and therefore not a needed service. For recipients to make an autonomous decision, they should be informed of the third-party influences on the provision of occupational therapy services.

Sometimes ethical dilemmas cannot be avoided. An ethical dilemma is created when two or more moral principles are in conflict. Moral principles in conflict can be beneficence (doing what is best), autonomy (right to self-determination), justice (distribution of benefits and burdens), and nonmaleficence (causing no harm). When an ethical dilemma occurs, it is best to gather information prior to making a decision. Answer these simple questions:

(1) What is the dilemma?

(2) What principles are in conflict?

(3) What values are in conflict?

(4) Do I have all the facts I need to make a decision?

(5) What are my options?

(6) What are the potential outcomes of the options?

After you have answered these questions, take the appropriate action(s).

Some sample dilemmas to be used as points for group discussion follow. What would you do in each situation?

Dilemmas

(1) What is the concern when the occupational therapy practitioner has a relationship with a patient and the occupational therapy practitioner is pressed to increase the number of billable units for assessment by discharging the longer-term patients from treatment? The occupational therapy practitioner is told to add new patients in need of the more costlier assessment as quickly as possible.

(2) What is the concern when the occupational therapy practitioner working in low-income environments has to decide who may receive adaptive equipment when that equipment is distributed free of charge, yet the OT manager is told to hold down costs?

(3) What is the concern when a clinical educator in a teaching hospital that trains Level II fieldwork students, because of his or her productivity requirements, does not have as much time as he or she thinks is necessary to shadow students? Students are expected to be productive at an early stage in the fieldwork experience.

(4) What is the concern when the mission of a contract therapy service is to make as much profit as legally as possible, and occupational therapy practitioners are required on short notice to increase services to a population many believe are not in need of occupational therapy?

(5) What is the concern when there is an increase in the number of noncertified personnel working with patients? Although the company says they are not doing skilled therapy their services are still billed as OT. The noncertified personnel work in the evenings and on weekends without an OT on site to supervise. The OT supervisor has a beeper and may be called by the noncertified personnel should the need arise.

(6) What is the concern when there is an increased need to use aides, trained on the job, whose cost are included in the per diem rate in the performance of range of motion activities? The occupational therapy practitioner raises concerns regarding training these individuals and sees what he or she is doing as "giving the store away." How much training is too much training?

(7) What is the concern when a new graduate has accepted a position with a contract company in a nonlicensing state? The new graduate has failed the AOTCB certification exam. The contract company does not share this information with the employer when placing the new graduate. The new graduate signs his or her notes OTR or COTA, which you as the supervisor think means he or she has passed the exam. For the last two months, the occupational therapy supervisor has been co-signing the new graduate's notes.

(8) What is the concern when some facilities are using broad guidelines that restrict the recipient of services from having a variety of care and choices? Occupational therapy is not always included in these choices. Physicians are reluctant to be part of an ad hoc system of rationing and feel it is the professional responsibility of OT to become one of the choices they can select. Occupational therapy practitioners feel it is "unprofessional to advertise themselves."

These are just a few examples of ethical dilemmas seen by occupational therapy practitioners working in the managed care environment. As dilemmas arise, it is best to look to the

Code and Core Values as action guides. The provision of services in a virtuous manner is a statement of commitment to the best interest of the recipient of service. ▼

REFERENCES

American Occupational Therapy Association. (1993). Core values and attitudes of occupational therapy practice. *American Journal of Occupational Therapy, 47*(12), 1085–1086.

American Occupational Therapy Association. (1994). Occupational therapy code of ethics. *American Journal of Occupational Therapy, 48*(11), 1037–1038.

Council on Ethical and Judicial Affairs, American Medical Association. (1995). Ethical issues in managed care. *Journal of the American Medical Association, 273*(4), 330–335.

Engelhardt, H. T., & Rie, M. A. (1988). Morality for the medical-industrial complex: A code of ethics for the mass marketing of health care. *New England Journal of Medicine, 319*(16), 1086–1089.

Perspectives on Managed Care

Occupational therapy practitioners nationwide are feeling the effects of managed care on the delivery of occupational therapy services. Managed care is a fundamentally different way of providing health care treatment. There are variations depending on the model employed, but managed care seeks to do precisely what the words imply: "manage care" and reduce unneeded or unnecessary care, thus containing costs.

What has been the impact of managed care on occupational therapy practitioners and how they practice? What will be the future for the profession, given that managed care is here to stay? What should practitioners do to best position themselves for success in this environment? If you have asked yourself questions like these, you are not alone!

AOTA decided to contact a number of prominent practitioners to find out how managed care has affected the way they practice and to learn their perspective on what the key issues are that individual practitioners and the profession as a whole need to address. The practitioners whom AOTA contacted were very candid in their responses. Overall, they believe that the environment offers many opportunities for practitioners to assume even more significant roles in providing rehabilitation services. Here is some of what they had to say:

"I think that what we have to do is design a treatment plan for our profession," said Yolanda Bruce Brooks, PsyD, OTR, a clinical psychologist in private practice who teaches at Texas Woman's University school of occupational therapy in Dallas. "We need to help ourselves do what we help clients do: adapt and change to new circumstances. As with our clients, the first place one starts is with outlook and mind-set. We must adopt a new attitude and approach. We have to accept that the way health care services were once delivered no longer exists. We have to accept that health care is a business."

Brooks believes practitioners need to educate themselves about the business aspects of health care, including marketing. Practitioners must also target managed care entities and third-party payers with messages about the value of occupational therapy. Practitioners should also consider becoming case managers for managed care companies. Consumers also need to be made aware of the value of occupational therapy, according to Brooks, because if they do, the third-party payers will follow suit.

Brooks see occupational therapy returning to its roots, with an emphasis on wellness, function, and holistic, proactive approaches to treatment. "What are the practice areas where occupational therapy practitioners can be of service?" she asks. "It's all of them!"

L. Randy Strickland, EdD, OTR/L, who is regional rehabilitation director for Hillhaven, Inc., headquartered in Louisville, Kentucky, has held numerous leadership positions in the association, including serving as chairperson of the Directions for the Future task force. He reflected on some of the positive impacts of managed care on occupational therapy—impacts managed care has had on virtually the entire health care industry.

"Changes in payment for services are helping us to think about what we are doing and why," said Strickland. "Managed care is helping us to think about what is a skilled service, who the best person is to provide the service needed, and what is the most cost-effective treatment."

Strickland doesn't deny, however, that managed care creates challenges for practitioners. Realistically, practitioners are no longer in control of determining the frequency and duration of treatment. Situations may occur that raise concerns about whether clients are receiving the best care. In those cases, he suggests a three-step approach.

▼ First, practitioners must determine what the client's needs are and prioritize them, especially taking into consideration safety issues such as, "Can my patient function safely in bathing or transferring in the bathroom?" Then, practitioners have to ask if the therapy provided is the most cost-effective use of the therapist's or assistant's time based on determining what the client needs.

▼ Second, if the time allotted for patient treatment is not enough to guarantee the client's ability to function safely, the practitioner needs to approach the payer with documented information about what the patient needs and what level of treatment will ensure the best outcome.

▼ Third, if the payer does not agree with the practitioner's judgment, then the practitioner needs to pursue the matter at the next highest level.

Strickland believes the future is bright if occupational therapy can, as Brooks pointed out, adopt a proactive approach based on demonstrated outcomes. Practitioners do need to understand how the service delivery system works and become a part of it. Practitioners must not accept what the systems dictates and provide undocumented treatment, for instance, to make up the difference in what the practitioner determines the patient needs.

"One has to know what it costs to provide a particular service and be able to reconcile that with what is being paid," said Diane McCarthy, MS, OTR/L, who works for Medbridge, Inc, in Arlington, Virginia. "It sounds very basic, and to people who work in a small business or who are familiar with the financial aspects of how an occupational therapy department works, it may be old hat. But practitioners have to know how to balance the cost of what a patient receives with what the payer will reimburse and then plan treatment accordingly."

McCarthy discussed how essential it is to develop rapport with case managers and benefits coordinators. One-on-one education of the people who are responsible for adjudicating the application of health care resources is essential. It is McCarthy's observation that where one will find flexibility in payment, length of treatment, and other areas, is in the hands of the people responsible for monitoring patient care for the payers. In addition, McCarthy stressed the importance of businesses and companies being part of provider networks.

Like Brooks, McCarthy also discussed how important it is to help make patients aware of possible limitations in coverage for occupational therapy services. If patients are aware of what their insurance will and will not pay for, they are in a position to advocate for what they need, including coverage for occupational therapy.

When commenting on the most profound impacts managed care has had on occupational therapy, Jim King, OTR, CHT, of HealthSouth Sports Medicine and Rehabilitation Center in Waco, Texas, cited many positives and many challenges. Among the positive impacts he cited are the increased focus on customer service and outcomes, the ongoing effort to develop algorithms for treatment and critical pathways, and increased productivity. Among the challenges managed care presents are morale issues caused by downsizing and the decrease in "hands-on" time practitioners have with their clients.

King believes "managed care provides an opportunity for the profession and should be viewed as such. We will have an opportunity to show once and for all the legitimacy of occupational therapy as a cost-effective method of reducing the overall cost of treatment." Along with the others AOTA contacted, King mentioned the need to focus on the business aspects of the profession. Practitioners have to manage the cost per visit, and find ways to see greater numbers of patients while still achieving excellent outcomes. In addition, King mentioned the need to continue to devise empirically supported treatment algorithms, and the need to learn case management, negotiation, and conflict resolution skills to assist in working with payers.

Linda Niemeyer, OTR, is research coordinator at Rehab Technology Works, in San Bernardino, California. Like many practitioners in California, she has been immersed in managed care for some time! Overall, Niemeyer thinks there are four areas of critical concern with regard to managed care and occupational therapy: (1) capitation, case rates, and prospective payment; (2) accountability for functional outcomes; (3) critical pathways; and (4) resource management.

"If the capitation rate is not adequate to cover the cost of care, the provider loses money, and this may lead to providers refusing to take the more difficult and costly cases," she observed. "It could also lead to sacrificing quality of care. The problem is that the Medicare prospective payment system for inpatient rehabilitation, which uses DRGs to determine the level of payment, does not adequately capture resource use for rehabilitation patients. For example, functional status at admission—as opposed to diagnosis—has a stronger association with length-of-stay and cost.

"A better classification system would group patients based on functional status," she points out. "What better role for occupational therapy practitioners than to help develop meaningful and reliable measures of functional status and to use this toward developing classification systems for rehabilitation where capitation and prospective payment do not penalize either the patient or the provider."

Niemeyer also pointed out that in all segments of the health care industry, insurance companies are now commonly tracking the course of care and outcomes on computer data-bases. These companies are paying attention to the track records of providers, and those providers who are not producing predetermined outcomes within a predetermined cost framework may be excluded from managed care contracts. "Occupational therapy practitioners can and must play a role in developing reliable and valid functional outcome measures, tracking outcomes and course of care in their own programs, and implementing continuous performance improvement based upon information gathered," said Niemeyer.

Closely related to this, occupational therapy practitioners can and must play a role in developing critical pathways for the patients they treat. An insurance company can pull from its database the typical course of care for a given type of patient and then compare those records with the performance of a given provider. They will tend not to contract with providers that deviate strongly from this standard. "Critical pathways based solely on billing codes may miss some of the aspects of a course of care," Niemeyer added. "Occupational therapy practitioners are the ones with the knowledge to develop critical pathways that reflect the true needs of the patient."

Finally, Niemeyer addressed the need for practitioners to play a role in making what might be hard decisions regarding allocation of resources. In other words, as others have also said, who is going to deliver care? How is it going to be delivered? And might this mean the greater use of certified assistants and aides?

Understanding the business side of health care; developing a proactive approach to dealing with managed care that includes educating payers and patients alike; participating in the process of defining established courses of treatment—these are the ways practitioners are successfully "managing" managed care! ▼

107

Accommodating Fieldwork in a Managed Care Environment

INTRODUCTION

Managed care affects practitioners who provide fieldwork supervision for OT and OTA students, students who are entering the managed care environment for their fieldwork experience, and academic educators who provide students with the information and skills to help prepare them to function effectively in this type of practice environment.

The following information is intended to assist academic educators, fieldwork educators, and OT/OTA students in understanding the impact of managed care on fieldwork education. Topics include

(1) the impact of managed care on fieldwork;

(2) the commitment to training students;

(3) suggestions for redesigning fieldwork experiences for students that reduce the stress on staff;

(4) school and clinic partnerships;

(5) an example of a successful Level II fieldwork plan in a managed care environment; and

(6) background information and additional resources.

THE IMPACT OF MANAGED CARE ON FIELDWORK

One of the most obvious signs of the impact of managed care on clinical education has been the increased reluctance of some therapists to supervise students. This is influenced by the reorganization of the clinical education settings away from the traditional models and the increased focus on staff productivity. This has especially affected the willingness and motivation of sites to develop new student programs and has contributed to the current state of decreased fieldwork sites. The following represent the major concerns of the fieldwork educator in a managed care environment:

- ▼ Staff are concentrating on achieving treatment quotas. Staff are being pressured to meet treatment hour requirements. Frequently their continued employment depends on maintaining a specified number of units of treatment per day. Maintaining work demands is presumed to be in conflict with training students.

- ▼ Staff reductions are causing constant adjustments to changes in staff responsibilities. As hospitals and other treatment centers are struggling to stay in business, staff numbers have been critically reduced. Many departments, including occupational therapy departments, have had to redefine and realign job responsibilities. Staff are feeling pressured to learn new duties, adjust to new department structures, and assume additional responsibilities. Training students can seem to be too time consuming.

- ▼ Patients are frequently more acutely ill as they enter treatment and do not stay as long in treatment as they did before managed care. Fieldwork educators are adjusting to the shorter lengths of stay that patients have in treatment. They often are reluctant to have students work with patients in such fragile states of their illness.

- ▼ Student programming seems to be the most expendable to ease the pressures of new or changed responsibilities. Fieldwork educators and/or facility administrators have made decisions to discontinue student training programs to ease the pressures left by managed care. Managed care does not pay for student training.

- ▼ Staff commitment to student training is challenged. While fieldwork educators continue to recognize the importance of student training, mastering the work environment has a greater priority for them.

THE COMMITMENT TO TRAINING STUDENTS

Many OT practitioners are envisioning the occupational therapist of tomorrow as a consultant, administrator, or case manager. In clinical education, students are still learning the basic technical skills with less focus on the professional skills. In a managed care environment, it is critical for students to learn leadership roles with less emphasis on the basic skills. Clinical educators will also have to make a commitment to training students. OT/OTA practitioners should:

- ▼ Decide to train students. If allowed by the facility, fieldwork educators may continue to support their profession by offering student training programs. Once a decision to train students is made, fieldwork educators' next task is to problem-solve the best ways to train students in their facility without allowing the training to become extremely burdensome to the staff.

- ▼ Identify how students can be involved in patients with managed care. Fieldwork educators need to be aggressive in providing opportunities for students to learn how to treat patients under the pressures of managed care. Students can be strong contributors to the treatment processes with a carefully designed training program.

- ▼ Review and revise the model of training and supervision you have been using. It is important to understand that the traditional method of one student to one therapist supervision may need to be changed. Explore the possibility of using other facility personnel to assist with the supervision of the students. Many hands-on tasks can be taught by other staff (e.g., transfers, coleading groups). The use of other staff helps the student learn the importance of collaboration among disciplines. In a managed care environment collaboration and shared responsibilities among staff are essential.

- ▼ Consider using alternative models for fieldwork described in *OT Week* and discussed in COE meetings. Models such as group supervision, OT and OTA partnership, on-site faculty supervision, weekly OT supervision with daily supervision provided by a non-OT might be considered. Whichever model chosen needs to be appropriate for the fieldwork educator's facility, safety of the patients, and school requirements.

- ▼ Work with the OT schools and councils to help make changes in your fieldwork requirements. Fieldwork coordinators and school councils are strong resources for helping OT educators brainstorm ways to make changes in student training programs. The Education Department at AOTA, regional fieldwork consultants, and COE Fieldwork Issues Committee members are also good resources for helping OT educators be creative and aggressive in revising student training programs.

SUGGESTIONS FOR REDESIGNING FIELDWORK EXPERIENCES FOR STUDENTS THAT REDUCE THE STRESS ON STAFF

Developing or continuing student programs in this "change environment" requires a shift in thinking and a redesigning of the clinical education experience. The potential clinical educator must consider innovative models of fieldwork in terms of the type of supervision, the student's schedule for both Level I and Level II fieldwork, and the type of setting or clinical experience that could be provided. Experienced fieldwork educators have been able to reduce the stress of the staff by using the following strategies:

- ▼ Shift much of the onus of learning to the student. Students are used to following a syllabus for learning. Once they are provided with an outline for fieldwork with weekly assignments, resources, and expectations, the students can become responsible for their own learning (e.g., they set up in-service training appointments, they make sure they are getting the training they need). The OT supervisor can check on the progress in weekly meetings with the student. It makes students more independent and is a nice transition from school to clinic, while reducing some of the pressure on the fieldwork educator.

▼ Clearly define in writing the students' weekly assignments. This is a time-consuming process at first, but it has many benefits. Students appreciate the information and feel more in control of their learning experience. It also serves as a helpful reminder for supervisors, enabling them to better support the students' learning experiences (see example).

▼ Define the people and resources for students to contact to gain knowledge or training in specific areas. In the orientation and again in the weekly expectations or resource listings, the people and literature resources available to the students need to be clearly defined with locations and phone numbers. If resources are presented in written form, the students can access them independently.

▼ Use many staff (OT and others) to teach specific skills (e.g., evaluations, documentation, community resources, supply inventory, use of modalities). The use of other (non-OT) staff promotes collaboration, respect for, and effective working relationships with other team members. The use of other disciplines to teach and train students also helps the students define who they are as OTs. The fieldwork educator and supervisor can use weekly meetings to discuss the role of OT and uniqueness and similarities of OT to other disciplines.

▼ Use group training and supervision as much as possible. The use of groups allows students to learn from each other and to explore many professional problems and issues that they will face as clinicians (e.g., problem-solving how to choose activities, blurred roles, managed care pressures, health care changes). The use of groups encourages students to reach out to peers for professional support and continued learning experiences.

▼ Keep individual supervision sessions short and well focused on issues that are related to that one student's performance. Collective student concerns can be discussed in group supervision. Individual sessions are needed with students to complete evaluations and deal with specific problems related to the individual student. Ask the student to establish an agenda.

▼ Shift your thinking about training from one-to-one supervision to more facilitative supervision that helps students to connect the experiences they are having. When the onus of learning is on the student, the fieldwork educator has the unique role of being able to enjoy the mentoring process of exploring the questions about the profession that students raise and struggle to find the answers with them. It becomes the basis for facilitating the students' socialization into the profession.

▼ Involve students in managed care activities (e.g., setting up aftercare plans, case management, efficacy studies, performance improvement studies). Fieldwork educators have an obligation to involve students in managed care activities as much as possible. When they become therapists, they will be involved in a managed care environment and they need all the experiences they can get while in training. They do not need to be protected from managed care problems.

SCHOOL AND CLINIC PARTNERSHIPS

One of the most important relationships in clinical education is that between the school and the clinic. This is a collaborative relationship that is critical to this new health care environment. The schools have the obligation to teach students about managed care and its impact on health care. The fieldwork educators have the obligation to teach students about managed care and its impact on direct patient care.

Many schools are already creating supervisory expectations in the various settings with support from fieldwork educators. Many schools have already created supervisory partnerships for student training (faculty participating in student supervision) and have discussed group supervision models to prepare students for less one-on-one supervision. Many schools have incorporated fieldwork seminars into fieldwork experiences to help facilitate the students' success in fieldwork. Together, the schools and fieldwork educators are helping to mold the future of OT in a managed care environment.

▼ Schools have already begun to teach students about the impact of managed care in treatment. Faculty have actively gathered information about managed care and presented it to students in the classroom setting. It is the role of fieldwork educators to provide the learning modules for addressing managed care in the clinics. It is helpful for the clinics and the schools to share their information with each other at clinical council meetings or individually. The rapid changes in managed care make the communication exchanges vital.

▼ OT education programs have been innovative in creating supervisory partnerships for student training, and they are very strong resources for fieldwork educators to use in exploring new methods for creating student training experiences. Some schools have arranged faculty supervision models; others have been mentors for developing unique fieldwork experiences. Clinical councils have been resourceful in discussing alternative supervision models. Fieldwork coordinators have been strong resources for connecting fieldwork educators with similar questions about fieldwork with each other. The school and clinic partnerships are an essential ingredient in the successful training of our profession's future clinicians and researchers.

114

BELMONT CENTER FOR COMPREHENSIVE TREATMENT
PHILADELPHIA, PA
DAY PROGRAM FIELDWORK II

Overall Expectations

▼ Become an active part of treatment team.

▼ Achieve beginning-level competency in documentation (e.g., general assessment, SOAP notes, discharge notes, ADL evaluations, MVPT, treatment plans).

▼ Develop a minimum of 1 group, e.g., design, conduct independently.

▼ Conduct minimum of 2–3 groups independently.

▼ Colead or lead a minimum of 2 groups per day.

▼ Colead community meeting.

▼ Become knowledgeable in and comfortable with using group process in psychoeducational groups and activity-based group therapy.

▼ Develop strong basic repertoire of activities for use in treatment.

▼ Recognize how theory base is applied in treatment.

▼ Identify attributes of self as a therapist.

▼ Give a formal presentation of group(s) developed and run independently according to established criteria (see attached).

▼ Actively contribute to supervision.

▼ Become knowledgeable in working with a variety of managed health care companies.

▼ Be responsible for case management of 2–3 patients.

115

Rehabilitative Service Department

OCCUPATIONAL THERAPY

Baseline requirement per week for adult day program placements

WEEK I

▼ Orientation to FEW expectations, supervision model, weekly requirements.

▼ Orientation basic program, safety, keys, Code 22 (psych. emergency), Code 99 (medical emergency), fire (use firebox key).

▼ Set up SOAP Note review with OT supervisor, write first note.

▼ Observe adult day program (ADP) groups, community meeting.

▼ Complete self-evaluation.

▼ Identify groups in which you might like to be coleader.

▼ Set up meeting to review inpatient groups with OT supervisor.

WEEK II

▼ Orientation of ADP SOAP notes with OT fieldwork coordinator.

▼ Continue to observe treatment groups (including rotating through group[s] with which you will be working more permanently in ADP and inpatient groups).

▼ Closely observe 2 patients in ADP groups. Review charts of those patients.

▼ Complete 2 progress notes daily by the end of the week on patients with whom you worked or observed closely.

▼ Attend team meetings (Tuesday and Thursday 3:00–4:00 P.M.).

▼ Set up meeting with team members to discuss their responsibilities.

▼ Begin initial planning of group you will lead.

▼ Review intake procedure with OT supervisor.

▼ Begin work in 1–2 inpatient groups as coleader.

▼ Schedule supervision sessions.

WEEK III

▼ Rotate through scheduled groups—taking a more active leadership role.

▼ Continue to work with/observe individual patients in groups.

▼ Observe intakes with as many staff as possible.

▼ Practice intake procedure on others, if possible.

▼ Attend team meetings.

▼ Write SOAP progress notes on 2–3 patients daily.

▼ Plan group you will lead.

▼ Set up in-service with OT fieldwork coordinator to discuss activity group process.

▼ Set up in-service to discuss managed care with fieldwork coordinator.

▼ Set up in-service to review evaluation processes—MVPT, ACL, Kohlman with OT supervisor.

WEEK IV

▼ Observe at least one intake.

▼ Continue working with individual patients.

▼ Continue in assigned groups with increased planning and leadership.

▼ Write progress notes on 3–4 patients daily.

▼ Finalize plans for beginning own group.

▼ Take over responsibility for 2–3 ongoing groups.

▼ Assume case management responsibilities for 1 patient.

▼ Set up inservice to review family meetings.

WEEK V

▼ Begin leading own group.

▼ Pick up new patients (intakes).

▼ Continue to write progress notes.

▼ Set up in-service with social service department to review community service supports available for ADP patients.

▼ Add continuing case management.

▼ Observe family meeting.

WEEK VI

▼ Continue progress note writing.

▼ Schedule field visit, if desired.

▼ Think about final presentation.

▼ Consider dropping inpatient group.

▼ Mid-term evaluation.

▼ Identify other experiences you would like.

▼ Continue autonomy and responsibilities in individual sessions, treatment teams and treatment groups (i.e., processing) pick up additional groups, if appropriate, actively contribute to team meetings, documentation).

▼ Field visit, if desired.

▼ Consider changing groups.

▼ Begin preparing final presentation.

▼ Conduct family meeting/contact.

WEEK VII–XII

▼ Continue autonomy and responsibilities in ADP and inpatient groups.

▼ Plan final presentation.

▼ Final presentation will be held in last 2 weeks of affiliation.

118

Rehabilitative Services Department

SELF-EVALUATION AND LEARNING OBJECTIVES

Name: _____

Week of: _____

Areas of strength for use in this fieldwork.

1. _____

2. _____

3. _____

4. _____

5. _____

Areas needing improvement/fears associated with this fieldwork experience:

1. _____

2. _____

3. _____ 119

4. _____

5. _____

Learning objectives for this fieldwork experience:

1. _____

2. _____

3. _____

4. _____

5. _____

What do you expect from your supervisor:

FINAL PRESENTATION

To be presented within the final 2 weeks of fieldwork to the ADP treatment team.

TOPIC: Present the group or groups you developed covering the following information:

- ▼ Rationale for choosing particular type of group or topics

- ▼ OT theory base used in developing group

- ▼ Goals of group

- ▼ Description of group

- ▼ Format of group

- ▼ Types of patients who would benefit from group

- ▼ Outcomes of group

- ▼ Patient response to group

- ▼ Materials used in group

- ▼ Recommendations for continuation of group(s)

- ▼ Must supply protocol(s) of group or groups as handouts during presentation

ORIENTATION CHECKLIST

1. Orientation to Hospital (check all that apply)
   ____ Adult day program (ADP)
   ____ Older adult day program
   ____ Inpatient tour of hospital including units
   ____ Introduction to staff
   ____ Review of maps

2. Orientation to Pincus
   ____ Introduction to RSD staff
   ____ Tour of treatment areas
   ____ Location of bathrooms

3. Orientation to Keys
   ____ Common key to units
   ____ Key to student office
   ____ Key to treatment areas
   ____ Firebox key

4. Phone Usage
   ____ Review of voice mail
   ____ List of important phone numbers

5. Supervision Model

6. Fieldwork Responsibilities
   ____ Goals
   ____ Assignments
   ____ Week-by-week schedule
   ____ Activity schedules

7. Tables of Organization
   ____ Hospital
   ____ Day program
   ____ RSD

8. Philosophy
   ____ Belmont
   ____ RSD (rehabilitative service department)
   ____ OT (occupational therapy)
   ____ RT (recreational therapy)
   ____ MT (music therapy)
   ____ AT (art therapy)
   ____ PD (psychodrama)
   ____ Vision
   ____ Values

9. Code 22 Psych. Emergency
   ____ Explanation
   ____ Role of therapist during a code

10. Code 99 Medical Emergency
   ____ Explanation
   ____ Role of therapist during a code

11. Safety and Infection Control (see attached information)

12. Severe Weather or Weather Emergency (see attached)

13. Dress Code

14. Patient Supervision

Submitted by Nancy Beck, MA,OTR/L, Director, Adult Day Program, Rehabilitative Services, Belmont Center for Comprehensive Treatment, Philadelphia, PA

BACKGROUND INFORMATION AND ADDITIONAL RESOURCES

A. Regional Fieldwork Consultants

An important group of volunteers who serve as a link between AOTA's national office and the grassroots membership is the regional fieldwork consultant (RFWC) network. These are current, active fieldwork educators who have been selected to represent AOTA on fieldwork matters in their particular regions. AOTA has carved out nine regions in the United States, each with its own consultant. These volunteer consultants are full-time practitioners who provide their expertise and present workshops to their constituents. Some of the workshop topics have been the fundamentals of supervision, clinical reasoning, multicultural aspects of fieldwork, OT/OTA fieldwork partnerships, and the how-to's of setting up clinical fieldwork programs. AOTA relies quite heavily on the consultants for mutual information exchange and updates from their regions on fieldwork happenings. Close attention is paid to states that AOTA identifies as underserved where there may be no occupational therapy educational programs and/or there are low ratios of occupational therapy practitioners to population.

AOTA members or others may contact AOTA's Fieldwork Education Program Manager, Christine Privott, MA, OTR/L, for guidance and help in interpreting the "essentials" of fieldwork. Faculty members, students, and practitioners involved in fieldwork may be seeking guidance on the failing student, the interpretation of the Fieldwork Evaluation Form, or to brainstorm innovative ideas for fieldwork. Hearing from and listening to individuals nationwide enables the fieldwork program manager to track trends and developments within the profession and direct members to appropriate, available, and useful resources.

B. Information Available from the AOTA Education Department

Information Packet for Developing Student Affiliations—OT/OTA
This is a packet of information for the clinical placement who is developing a new Level II fieldwork program for students.

The Guidelines for an Occupational Therapy Fieldwork Experience—Level I and Level II—1992 and 1993, respectively. These guidelines facilitate the interpretation of the *Essentials*. These guidelines are not official documents; however, they help determine optimal fieldwork practice arrangements and clarify requirements for successful completion of fieldwork.

Essentials and Guidelines for an Accredited Educational Program for the Occupational Therapist—1991—Updated and *Essentials and Guidelines for an Accredited Educational Program for the Occupational Therapy Assistant—1991—Updated.* These *Essentials* are the "minimum standards of quality used in accrediting programs that prepare individuals to enter the occupational therapy profession" (page 1). They are included in *The Guide to Fieldwork Education* and the information packets for new fieldwork sites.

Fieldwork Data Form (AOTA, 1995). This form is used by clinical facilities to describe what their site has to offer regarding fieldwork. The schools keep this information on file for students and educators.

Student Evaluation of Fieldwork Experience (1995). This is the form that a majority of clinical placements use for the student to evaluate the fieldwork experience.

Members who wish to become more involved in fieldwork programming at the national and regional levels are invited to contact the AOTA Fieldwork Education Program Manager and check *OT Week, AJOT, OT Practice*, and *Special Interest Section Newsletters* for announcements. For information about volunteer opportunities through local or regional fieldwork councils, the academic program can be an excellent resource. State associations may also have student and fieldwork representation on their boards. Another viable option for exploring volunteer possibilities in fieldwork is to contact the RFWC network.

C. Information Available from AOTA Products

The Guide to Fieldwork Education—Commission on Education, Fieldwork Issues Committee, 1994. This is the recently revised in-depth guide to the many aspects of fieldwork. It is a useful fieldwork reference for OT education programs, the clinical sites, and students as it contains chapters on legal and ethical principles, supervision, sample forms, and current examples of fieldwork objectives for Level I and II (as it relates to the Fieldwork Evaluation Form) as well as sample student schedules.

123

Self-Paced Instruction for Clinical Education and Supervision (SPICES), 1991. This is a training model and video developed for supervisory training programs in the clinic. The workbook can be purchased by facilities as well as educational programs and used as part of their continuing education program for new and experienced OT supervisors of students. Each section is authored by a fieldwork specialist and includes experimental exercises and videotape case studies. The content includes assessing readiness for a student program, developing and understanding objectives, learning about the developmental needs of students, and developing clinical reasoning skills.

Occupational Therapy: Transition from Classroom to Clinic—Physical Disability Fieldwork Applications (Smith, 1994). This book is for fieldwork supervisors and students to help bridge the gap between academics and practice. The workbook format is very useful in the classroom and clinic.

Fieldwork Evaluation for the Occupational Therapist (AOTA, 1987) and *Fieldwork Evaluation for the Occupational Therapy Assistant Students* (AOTA, 1983). These are the standard assessment tools for occupational therapy students. Most clinical placements and schools advocate the use of these evaluations for their students.

The Reliable Source (formerly *OT Source*), a computer software program available from AOTA, is also a worthwhile resource to access fieldwork sites (as listed in the OT Fieldwork Centers book) and fieldwork bibliographical information.

Some issues of the *Education Special Interest Section Newsletter,* published quarterly by AOTA, also include articles on fieldwork. Recent topics in fieldwork discussed in these newsletters have been fieldwork and the Americans with Disabilities Act, innovative fieldwork models, and mental health fieldwork. EDSIS members receive the newsletter free. Others may purchase individual copies through AOTA Products.

124

Managed Care
Reference Information

CONTENTS

MANAGED CARE PERIODICALS

The following is a compilation of journals and other publications that contain information related to managed care.

This list is by no means comprehensive and does not in any way represent the endorsement of AOTA. The listing is for informational purposes only.

Publications Related to Managed Care

TITLE: AAPPO (American Association of Preferred Provider Organizations)*

PUBLISHER: Health Care Communications, Inc.
1 Bridge Plaza
Fort Lee, NJ 07024

201-947-5545
201-947-8406 (Fax)

FREQUENCY/PRICE: Published bimonthly; $50/year

COVERAGE/LEVEL OF KNOWLEDGE: Highlights research and trends within managed health care.

TITLE: AARP Bulletin

PUBLISHER: American Association of Retired Persons
601 E Street, N.W.
Washington, DC 20049

202-434-2277

FREQUENCY/PRICE: Published 11 times per year; free to members

COVERAGE/LEVEL OF KNOWLEDGE: Includes current news from the executive branch, Congress, the courts, regulatory agencies, and state legislatures. Reports on Washington activities and national trends that have a bearing on the lives of older people.

TITLE: Advance for OTs

PUBLISHER: Merion Publications
650 Park Avenue West
King of Prussia, PA 19406

610-265-7812
610-265-8971 (Fax)

FREQUENCY/PRICE: Published weekly; free

TITLE: AHA News

PUBLISHER: American Hospital Publishing, Inc.
737 N. Michigan Avenue, Suite 700
Chicago, IL 60611

312-440-6800

FREQUENCY/PRICE: Published weekly; AHA members: $45/year; nonmembers: $100/year

COVERAGE/LEVEL OF KNOWLEDGE: Newsletter covering information on AHA activities and health care activities at the state and national level.

TITLE: Behavioral Healthcare Tomorrow

PUBLISHER: CentraLink
1110 Mar West Street, Suite E
Tiburon, CA 94920-9928

415-435-9848

FREQUENCY/PRICE: Published bimonthly. Individual rate: $65/year, $110/2 years; library/institutional rate: $95/year, $160/2 years

COVERAGE/LEVEL OF KNOWLEDGE: National dialogue journal on mental health and addiction treatment benefits and services in the era of managed care.

128

TITLE: Behavioral Health Management

PUBLISHER: MEDQUEST Communications, Inc.
P.O. Box 20179
Cleveland, OH 44120

216-522-9700
216-522-9707 (Fax)

FREQUENCY/PRICE: Published bimonthly; $50/year, $75/2 years, $95/3 years

COVERAGE/LEVEL OF KNOWLEDGE: Focuses on the best ways to adjust, live with, and profit from the new system (rapidly changing world of managed behavioral health care policy, rule's regulations, and prescribe protocols).

TITLE: BNA's Health Care Policy Report

PUBLISHER: The Bureau of National Affairs, Inc.
1231 25th Street, N.W.
Washington, DC 20037-1197

202-452-4200

FREQUENCY/PRICE: Published weekly; $716/year

COVERAGE/LEVEL OF KNOWLEDGE: Newsletter covering information on health care policy at the state and national level.

TITLE: BNA's Managed Care Reporter

PUBLISHER: The Bureau of National Affairs, Inc.
1231 25th Street, N.W.
Washington, DC 20037-1197

202-452-4200

FREQUENCY/PRICE: Published weekly; $595/year

COVERAGE/LEVEL OF KNOWLEDGE: Newsletter covering a range of important issues facing the managed care industry.

TITLE: BNA's Medicare Report

PUBLISHER: The Bureau of National Affairs, Inc.
1231 25th Street, NW
Washington, DC 20037-1197

202-452-4200

FREQUENCY/PRICE: Published weekly; $688/year

COVERAGE/LEVEL OF KNOWLEDGE: Newsletter covering information on Medicare and health care policy at the state and national level.

TITLE: Business & Health

PUBLISHER: Medical Economics Subscriber Services Dept.
Business & Health
P.O. Box 3090
Denville, NJ 07834

800-432-4570

FREQUENCY/PRICE: Published monthly; $99/year

COVERAGE/LEVEL OF KNOWLEDGE: Magazine addressing a broad range of public policy and worksite issues, including health system reform, disability, health promotion and disease prevention, maternal and child health, retirees and older workers, mental health, public and private partnerships, and quality purchasing.

TITLE: Caring

PUBLISHER: National Association for Home Care
519 C Street, N.E.
Washington, DC 20002-5809

202-547-7424
202-547-3590 (Fax)

FREQUENCY/PRICE: Published monthly; $45/year

COVERAGE/LEVEL OF KNOWLEDGE: Contains articles, special sections, and departments covering national and international aspects of the home care field.

TITLE: Case Manager

PUBLISHER: Mosby-Year Book, Inc.
11830 Westline Industrial Drive
St Louis, MO 63146-3318

800-453-4351 or 314-453-4351

FREQUENCY/PRICE: Published 5 times a year; $30/year

COVERAGE/LEVEL OF KNOWLEDGE: The business and professional publication of the Individual Case Management Association.

TITLE: Clear News

PUBLISHER: Council on Licensure, Enforcement, and Reimbursement
201 West Short Street, Suite 401
Lexington, KY 40507

606-231-1892
606-231-1943 (Fax)

FREQUENCY/PRICE: Published quarterly; no cost/call to put name on mailing list

COVERAGE/LEVEL OF KNOWLEDGE: Newsletter containing information on licensure at the state level.

TITLE: GAO Publications

PUBLISHER: U.S. General Accounting Office
P.O. Box 6015
Gaithersburg, MD 20884-6015

202-512-6000
301-258-4066 (Fax)

FREQUENCY/PRICE: Each day, GAO issues a list of newly available reports and testimony. To receive facsimile copies of the daily list or any list from the past 30 days, please call 301-358-4097. First copy free; $2 each additional copy.

COVERAGE/LEVEL OF KNOWLEDGE: Reports and testimonies on different subjects.

TITLE: Health Affairs

PUBLISHER: Project HOPE
7500 Old Georgetown Road, Suite 600
Bethesda, MD 20814

800-825-0061

FREQUENCY/PRICE: Published 5 times a year (Feb, May, July, Oct, Dec). Individuals: $45/year, $80/2 years, $120/3 years; institutions: $75/year, $135/2 years, $195/3 years

COVERAGE/LEVEL OF KNOWLEDGE: A multidisciplinary, peer-reviewed journal dedicated to the serious exploration of domestic and international health policy issues.

TITLE: Health Alliance Alert (formerly Health Business)*

PUBLISHER: Faulkner & Gray
Healthcare Information Center
(Subsidiary of Thomson Publishing Group)
1133 15th Street, N.W., Suite 450
Washington, DC 20005

202-828-4150
202-828-2532 (Fax)

FREQUENCY/PRICE: Published biweekly; $375/year

COVERAGE/LEVEL OF KNOWLEDGE: Covers financial and economic aspects of the U.S. health care industries.

TITLE: Healthcare Informatics

PUBLISHER: Health Data Analysis, Inc.
P.O. Box 2830
2902 Evergreen Parkway, Suite 100
Evergreen, CO 80439-9904

FREQUENCY/PRICE: Published monthly; $28/year

COVERAGE/LEVEL OF KNOWLEDGE: For health care information management (i.e. , computer systems).

TITLE: Health Line

PUBLISHER: American Political Network, Inc.
3129 Mount Vernon Avenue
Alexandria, VA 22305

703-518-4600
703-518-8703 (Fax)

FREQUENCY/PRICE: Daily; call for subscription rates

COVERAGE/LEVEL OF KNOWLEDGE: A daily news briefing on politics and policy, statelines, inside the industry, market watch, and access/quality/cost.

TITLE: Hospital's & Health Networks

PUBLISHER: American Hospital Publishing, Inc.
737 North Michigan Avenue
Chicago, IL 60611

312-440-6800

FREQUENCY/PRICE: Published bimonthly (24 times a year); $65/year

COVERAGE/LEVEL OF KNOWLEDGE: Covers information pertinent to hospitals and health networks. Regular departments include current affairs and inside track (executive management trends).

TITLE: Inquiry

PUBLISHER: Inquiry
P.O. Box 527
Glenview, IL 60025

708-724-9280

FREQUENCY/PRICE: Published quarterly. Individual rate: $50/year, $90/2 years; institutional rate: $70/year, $125/2 years

COVERAGE/LEVEL OF KNOWLEDGE: The journal of health care organization, provision, and financing.

TITLE: Journal of American Health Care Policy*

PUBLISHER: Faulkner & Gray, Inc.
Eleven Penn Plaza
New York, NY 10001-2006

800-535-8403

FREQUENCY/PRICE: Published bimonthly; $125/year

COVERAGE/LEVEL OF KNOWLEDGE: A national forum for the research findings and views of leading players in the U.S. health care system. Covers a broad scope of issues including access to and financing of medical care, economic patterns and impact, public health delivery systems, legal and ethical considerations, international system analysis and comparison, regulatory analysis, and emerging ideas and concepts from the public and private sectors.

TITLE: Journal of Practical Psychiatry and Behavioral Health

PUBLISHER: Williams & Wilkins
P.O. Box 23291
Baltimore, MD 21203-9990

800-638-6423
410-528-4312 (Fax)

FREQUENCY/PRICE: Published bimonthly. Individual rate: $73/year; institutional rate: $103/year

COVERAGE/LEVEL OF KNOWLEDGE: Contains news about scientific and clinical advances, reports on major professional meetings, continuing education, student assignments, reference/citation for research, trends in research and treatment. Has a regular column on managed care.

133

TITLE: Journal of Rehab Management

PUBLISHER: Allied Health Care Publications
4676 Admiralty Way, Suite 202
Marina del Rey, CA 90292

310-306-2206
310-301-3329 (Fax)

FREQUENCY/PRICE: Published bimonthly; call for subscription rates

COVERAGE/LEVEL OF KNOWLEDGE: Contains information on the rehabilitation industry.

TITLE: Managed Care*

PUBLISHER: Stezzi Communications, Inc.
301 Oxford Valley Road, Suite 603B
Yardley, PA 19067

215-321-6663
215-321-6677 (Fax)

FREQUENCY/PRICE: Published monthly; $72/year

COVERAGE/LEVEL OF KNOWLEDGE: Advises physicians in managed care on the conduct of their careers. Informs them of their rapidly changing options and opportunities.

TITLE: Managed Care Medicine*

PUBLISHER: Health Care Communications, Inc.
1 Bridge Plaza, Suite 350
Fort Lee, NJ 07024

201-947-5545
201-947-8406 (Fax)

FREQUENCY/PRICE: Published bimonthly; $95/year

COVERAGE/LEVEL OF KNOWLEDGE: Focuses on the business side of medicine.

TITLE: Managed Care Outlook

PUBLISHER: Capitol Publications, Inc.
1101 King Street, Suite 444
Alexandria, VA 22314-2968

800-655-5597

FREQUENCY/PRICE: Published biweekly; $439/year

COVERAGE/LEVEL OF KNOWLEDGE: The insider's business briefing on managed health care.

TITLE: Managed Care Quarterly*

PUBLISHER: Aspen Publishers, Inc.
200 Orchard Ridge Drive
Gaithersburg, MD 20878

301-417-7500
301-417-7550 (Fax)

FREQUENCY/PRICE: Published quarterly; $84/year

TITLE: Managed Care Week*

PUBLISHER: Atlantic Information Services, Inc.
1050 17th Street, NW, Suite 480
Washington, DC 20036

202-775-9008 or 800-521-4323
202-331-9542 (Fax)

FREQUENCY/PRICE: Published 45 times/year; call for subscription rates ($409–$502/year)

COVERAGE/LEVEL OF KNOWLEDGE: Timely news of HMOs, PPOs, POS plans, and innovative managed care arrangements.

TITLE: Managed Healthcare News*

PUBLISHER: Advanstar Communications, Inc.
1 East First Street
Duluth, MN 55082

800-346-0085

FREQUENCY/PRICE: Published monthly; $59/year

COVERAGE/LEVEL OF KNOWLEDGE: Directed toward health care benefits managers, managed health care organizations, providers of health care services. Covers issues of concern for managers responsible for controlling employee health care costs and quality, news, benefits and management, legislative and regulatory issues, utilization patterns, and pharmaceutical trends.

TITLE: Managed Medicare & Medicaid News (formerly Health Care Reform Week)

PUBLISHER: United Communications Group
11300 Rockville Pike, Suite 1100
Rockville, MD 20852-3030

800-929-4824 ext 223

FREQUENCY/PRICE: Published weekly (48 times/year); call for subscription rates

COVERAGE/LEVEL OF KNOWLEDGE: Newsletter containing information on managed care and health care reform.

TITLE: Medicare & Medicaid Guide

PUBLISHER: Commerce Clearing House
4025 West Peterson Avenue
Chicago, IL 60646

800-835-5224
800-224-8299 (Fax)

FREQUENCY/PRICE: Published weekly

COVERAGE/LEVEL OF KNOWLEDGE: Contains the Medicare and Medicaid laws and regulations, HCFA manuals.

TITLE: Modern Healthcare*

PUBLISHER: Crain Communications, Inc.
965 East Jefferson Avenue
Detroit, MI 48207-3185

800-678-9595

FREQUENCY/PRICE: Published weekly; $110/year

COVERAGE/LEVEL OF KNOWLEDGE: Contains information on health care management. Regular columns include news, technology, financial and legal briefs, new products, literature and professional exchange.

TITLE: NAMI Advocate

PUBLISHER: National Alliance for the Mentally Ill
2101 Wilson Boulevard, Suite 302
Arlington, VA 22201-3008

703-524-9094

FREQUENCY/PRICE: Published monthly; $25/year

COVERAGE/LEVEL OF KNOWLEDGE:

TITLE: NARA News

PUBLISHER: National Association of Rehabilitation Agencies
11250-8 Roger Bacon Drive, Suite 8
Reston, VA 22090

703-437-4377
703-435-4390 (Fax)

FREQUENCY/PRICE: Published bimonthly; subscription is by membership to NARA

COVERAGE/LEVEL OF KNOWLEDGE: Contains news information pertinent to rehabilitation agencies.

TITLE: NARF Rehab Report

PUBLISHER: National Association of Rehabilitation Facilities
P.O. Box 17675
Washington, DC 20041

703-648-9300
703-648-0346 (Fax)

FREQUENCY/PRICE: Free for members

TITLE: Part B News

PUBLISHER: United Communications Group
11300 Rockville Pike, Suite 1100
Rockville, MD 20852-3030

800-929-4824 ext 223
301-816-8945 (Fax)

FREQUENCY/PRICE: Published biweekly (24 times/year); $446/year

COVERAGE/LEVEL OF KNOWLEDGE: Independent news pertaining to Medicare Part B.

TITLE: Physician's Managed Care Report*

PUBLISHER: American Health Consultants
3525 Piedmont Road, N.E.
Building Six, Suite 400
Atlanta, GA 30305

404-262-7436 or 800-688-2421 (subscriber services)

FREQUENCY/PRICE: Published monthly; $289/year

COVERAGE/LEVEL OF KNOWLEDGE: Contains information on physician-hospital alliances, group structures, integration, contract strategies, capitation, case management, and HMO-PPO trends.

TITLE: Physician's Payment Update

PUBLISHER: American Health Consultants
3525 Piedmont Road, N.E.
Building Six, Suite 400
Atlanta, GA 30305

404-262-7436 or 800-688-2421 (subscriber services)

FREQUENCY/PRICE: Published monthly; $309/year or $824/3 years

COVERAGE/LEVEL OF KNOWLEDGE: Newsletter containing information on reimbursement and coding issues.

TITLE: Psychiatric Practice & Managed Care

PUBLISHER: Managed Care Services
American Psychiatric Association
1400 K Street, N.W.
Washington, DC 20005

800-343-4671
202-682-6348 (Fax)

FREQUENCY/PRICE: Published bimonthly; $55/year for APA members, $125/year nonmembers

COVERAGE/LEVEL OF KNOWLEDGE: Each issue features an article written by a guest editor, resources available to members, news updates, and reports from APA's components and district branches.

TITLE: Regulatory Affairs*

PUBLISHER: Regulatory Affairs Professional Society
12300 Twinbrook Parkway, Suite 630
Rockville, MD 20852

301-770-2920
301-770-2924 (Fax)

FREQUENCY/PRICE: Published quarterly; $120/year

COVERAGE/LEVEL OF KNOWLEDGE: Provides a worldwide forum for communication, education, and development for health care regulatory professionals in industry and government.

TITLE: Roll Call

PUBLISHER: Roll Call Associates
900 2nd Street, N.E.
Washington, DC 20002

202-289-4900

FREQUENCY/PRICE: Published biweekly (96 issues/year); $210/year or $370/2 years

COVERAGE/LEVEL OF KNOWLEDGE: Newsletter pertaining to activities on Capitol Hill.

TITLE: State ADM Reports

PUBLISHER: Intergovernmental Health Policy Project
2021 K Street, N.W., Suite 800
Washington, DC 20006

202-872-1445

FREQUENCY/PRICE: Published 10 times a year; $97/year

COVERAGE/LEVEL OF KNOWLEDGE: Covers important research and policy developments affecting mental health, alcoholism, and drug abuse programs within the 50 states.

TITLE: State Health Notes

PUBLISHER: Intergovernmental Health Policy Project
The George Washington University
2021 K Street, N.W., Suite 800
Washington, DC 20006

202-872-1445
202-785-0114 (Fax)

FREQUENCY/PRICE: Published biweekly (24 issues/year); $227/year or $147/year for nonprofit organizations, universities, and government employees

COVERAGE/LEVEL OF KNOWLEDGE: Newsletter containing information on health care news in the states.

BIBLIOGRAPHY

1. History

Cloutier, M. (1995). The evolution of managed care. *Trends in Health Care, Law & Ethics, 10*(1-2), 67–71.

> Ethical questions surrounding the managed care approach to health care and managed care's impact on the physician-patient relationship are examined. Physicians are required to resolve dilemmas of dual moral agency in their utilization decision in a managed care environment.

DeVita, E., & Emerson, G. (1995). The decline of the doctor-patient relationship. *American Health, 14*(5), 62–67.

Freund, D. A., & Hurley, R. E. (1995). Medicaid managed care: Contribution to issues of health reform. *Annual Review of Public Health, 16,* 473–495.

> This article examines the emergence of managed care in Medicaid from an alternative to the mainstream delivery system for many beneficiaries. It offers a definition that encompasses the broad spectrum of program manifestations and presents a brief historical perspective on the major eras of managed care in Medicaid. The major program prototypes are described and their contribution to enrollment growth is discussed. Research evidence is examined to address both operational issues and program impacts. Finally, we conclude with an appraisal of contemporary issues of importance and speculation on the next generation of Medicaid managed care programs with an eye toward how federal and state health care reform proposals will shape this future.

Gibson, D. (1989). Requisites for excellence: Structure and process in delivering psychiatric care. *Occupational Therapy in Mental Health, 9*(2), 27–52.

> Insurance regulations, strict admission and discharge criteria by managed care, and shortening length of stay in hospital psychiatry have created a need for the most efficient use of resources to provide the highest quality of care. Haddow (1986), a speaker at the National Association for Private Psychiatric Hospitals Conference, stated that various kinds of hospitals—short stay, long stay, high staff ratio, low staff ratio—all claim high quality of care. This article does not address costs, the value of one discipline or philosophy versus another, or varying length of stay; rather, it emphasizes the significance of role clarity, institutional requisites, and staff collaboration and communication in building and maintaining excellent quality of care.

Ginsburg, P. B. (1993). Expenditure limits and cost containment. *Inquiry, 30*(4), 389–399.

> The Clinton administration's proposal for health care reform would tie limits on premiums and, indirectly, provider payment rates to a national health care budget. This article analyzes provider rate setting and managed competition and discusses how they can be guided by expenditure limits. Particular attention is paid to health systems that include elements of both traditional fee-for-service insurance and organized systems of care.

Glossary of terms relating to managed care and capitation (1994). *Health System Leaders,* (Suppl.), 65–67.

Hettinger, J. (1995). Is it time to stop complaining about managed care and find ways to work within the system? AOTA President Mary Foto, OTR, FAOTA, believes it is. *OT Week, 9*(36), 19.

Kilbreth, E., & Cohen, A. B. (1993). Strategic choices for cost containment under a reformed U.S. health care system. *Inquiry, 30*(4), 372–388.

The Clinton administration health reform proposal would impose global spending limits to bring the rate of increase in health care spending into line with the consumer price index by 1999. This article examines cost containment strategies available to states and health plans under externally imposed revenue limits. Drawing on the experience of state and local regulatory agencies, private-sector managed care plans, and models in other countries, the authors contrast premium caps and provider rate setting as mechanisms to reduce growth in health care spending and briefly consider the system-level regulatory structures necessary to oversee and control aggregate health care spending.

Sheils, J. F., Lewin, L. S., & Haught, R. A. (1993). Potential public expenditures under managed competition. *Health Affairs (Millwood), 12*(Suppl.), 229–242.

This DataWatch estimates the public cost of providing universal coverage under a managed competition model. First, a uniform benefit package is specified; next, the lowest-cost premium for this coverage is estimated, based on average costs in a well-managed health maintenance organization. Based on these estimates, the costs of premium subsidies and tax revenue effects are determined. It is estimated that if coverage is extended to currently uninsured individuals using these estimates and assumptions, spending for those people will increase 73.9 percent over current levels. The authors estimate a net increase of $47.9 billion in 1993 health spending under a managed competition program with low patient cost sharing. This includes savings of $4.5 billion from wider use of managed care and $11.2 billion in administrative cost savings.

Staff, B. (1993). Employers give managed competition a new spin. *Business Health, 11*(11), 42, 44, 46 passim.

2. Organizational Perspective

Bennett, M. J. (1993). View from the bridge: Reflections of a recovering staff model HMO psychiatrist. *Psychiatry Quarterly, 64*(1), 45–75.

This article traces the origin and development of the mental health carve-out, relating it to its antecedents, and describing its three overlapping phases: utilization review, discounted fees, and network development and management. Part 2 describes the key concept of the continuum of care and the role of the case manager in monitoring a care episode. The article concludes by anticipating seven future trends and calling for mental health leadership to recognize and ally with the need to manage resources in a more rational and efficient manner.

Campbell, A. R., Vittinhoff, E., Morabito, D., Paine, M., Shagoury, C., Praetz, P., Grey, D., McAninch, J. W., & Schecter, W. P. (1995). Trauma centers in a managed care environment. *Journal of Trauma, 39*(2), 246–251.

Dragalin, D. (1994). How to evaluate managed care. *Journal of Health Care Benefits, 3*(4), 16–21.

Foto, M. (1993). Surviving managed care. *REHAB Management, 6*(1), 89–91.

Foto, M., & Swanson, G. (1993). Managed care: Integrated practice management. *REHAB Management, 6*(2), 107–108.

Hoge, M. A., Davidson, L., Griffith, E. E., Sledge, W. H., & Howenstine, R. A. (1994). Defining managed care in public-sector psychiatry. *Hospital Community Psychiatry, 45*(11), 1085–1089.

Although managed care is an established force in the private sector, there is growing interest and experimentation with this concept in the public sector. This interest has been generated by the increased demand for services, the shrinking resource base due to cutbacks in state budgets, and the fragmentation of care that has accompanied the shift from a centralized, hospital-based model to a decentralized, community-based model for treating individuals with serious mental illness. The authors present a functional analysis of managed care in the public sector. Drawing on their conceptualization of managed care, they outline a functional approach to evaluating the strengths and weaknesses of treatment systems, innovations such as privatization and capitation, and recent health care reform proposals.

Landress, H. J., & Bernstein, M. A. (1993). Managed care 101: An overview and implications for psychosocial rehabilitation services. *Psychosocial Rehabilitation Journal, 17*(2), 5–14.

Over the past decade, a variety of methods have been used by private insurers in an attempt to control rising health care expenditures. As health care costs continue to rise, states will increasingly turn to a variety of managed care methods to control Medicaid health and psychosocial rehabilitation agencies and the clients they serve. These changes include (1) the application of managed care methods to psychosocial rehabilitation, (2) more clients being medically case-managed, (3) specific agencies being designated to provide mental health services, (4) agencies incurring shared financial risk with states, (5) states contracting with intermediary agents, (6) the need for agencies to conduct self-inventories, and (7) services being bundled through health purchasing alliances.

McGarvey, M. R. (1995). The case for managed care. *Trends in Health Care, Law & Ethics, 10*(1–2), 45–46.

The benefits of managed care plans that emphasize pragmatic cost control approaches in combination with quality medical care are discussed. Physicians practicing in the managed care setting can reduce the number of unnecessary tests and treatments without compromising patient care.

Randall, V. R. (1994). Impact of managed care organizations on ethnic Americans and underserved populations. *Journal of Health Care for the Poor and Underserved, 5*(3), 224–236.

Managed care organizations (MCOs) use strict utilization review and financial risk-shifting to ensure that doctors and providers act as gatekeepers to health care services. The gatekeepers are assumed to continue to order necessary care and to eliminate only unnecessary care. However, significant potential for abuse exists. In fact, the very foundations on which MCO decisions are made are culturally biased, because they are based on information from largely middle-class, European-American, healthy males. Ultimately, MCOs will change the perceptions and expectations of

142

society regarding health care. These altered perceptions may be contrary to the needs of ethnic Americans, and without safeguards, could worsen existing disparities in health status.

Schauffler, H. H., & Rodriquez, T. (1993). Managed care for preventive services: A review of policy options. *Medical Care Review, 50*(2), 153–198.

Schuster, J. M. (1993). Managed care and mental health services: Lessons for health care providers. *American Journal of Medicine Quarterly, 8*(4), 200–203.

Managed health care has grown rapidly during the past decade and is likely to continue its expansion during the next several years. Psychiatric services have been subject to especially stringent efforts to control costs, including intensive utilization review and formation of provider networks that primarily use master-level professionals. Psychiatrists' responses to these changes have ranged from antagonistic to proactive. A thorough understanding of the impact of managed care upon psychiatry and of psychiatrists' responses can help providers in other medical specialties as they develop their own strategies to cope with the changing health care environment.

Staines, V. S. (1993). Potential impact of managed care on national health spending. *Health Affairs (Millwood), 12*(Suppl.), 248–257.

Illustrative estimates suggest that if all acute health care services were delivered through staff—or group-model health maintenance organizations (HMOs), national health spending might be almost 10 percent lower. If the delivery of all such services (except those now provided by staff- or group-model HMOs) were subject to utilization review arrangements incorporating precertification and concurrent review of inpatient care, spending might be 1 percent lower. The estimates assume no changes in the health care system apart from expansion of these two forms of managed care to cover all insured persons. They also assume that moving to universal managed care would produce a one-time drop in the level of national health spending with no subsequent effect on spending growth.

Terry, K. (1995). Has managed care rediscovered fee-for-service? *Medical Economy, 72*(13), 69–70, 75–76, 79–80.

Wanerman, L. (1993). Managed mental health for children and adolescents. *New Directions in Health Services, 59*, 13–26.

2.1 Change/Paradigm Shift

Bevilacqua, J. J. (1995). New paradigms, old pitfalls. *New Direction in Mental Health Services*, (66), 19–30.

Engelhard, C. L., & Childress, J. F. (1995). Caveat emptor: The cost of managed care. *Trends in Health Care, Law & Ethics, 10*(1-2), 11–14.

The extent to which managed care plans contain health care expenditures is examined, as are social-ethical concerns about managed care. There are costs to managed care plans that include a reduction of individual choice and autonomy.

Hettinger, J. (1995). New landscape, new models, new roles. *OT Week, 9*(42), 16–17.

Managed care has altered the health care landscape. Some experts believe OT practitioners need to change with it or risk being left behind.

Kolb, D. S., & Horowitz, J. L. (1995). Managing the transition to capitation. *Healthcare Financial Management, 49*(2), 64–69.

Although most experts believe that capitation and financial risk sharing among providers will become key components of the U.S. health care system, providers may not feel the full effect of this shift for several years. In the interim, providers must operate under an activity-based payment system that rewards them for the volume of patients seen, while preparing for the transition to a fixed, per capita payment system that will reward them for the efficiency with which services are provided. Preparation for the move to capitation will involve implementation of the systems necessary to negotiate managed care contracts, enhance quality and efficiency, and take responsibility for the health of a defined population.

Lamm, R. D. (1995). Managed care heresies. *Trends in Health Care, Law & Ethics, 10*(1–2), 15–18.

Eight heresies associated with the current state of health care in the U.S. that are also associated with the concept of managed care are presented and discussed. Policymakers must redefine and reconceptualize what keeps a society healthy.

Lee, F. C., & Cooper, T. M. (1994). Reengineering managed behavioral healthcare. *Behavioral Healthcare Tomorrow, 3*(2), 57–62.

Reengineering is an industrial method for rethinking and redesigning basic business processes to improve performance and lower cost. This article reviews basic principles of reengineering in the context of the evolving managed behavioral health care industry, defines 10 core processes for managed behavioral health care companies, and then illustrates how reengineering methods can be applied to two intermediate processes: manage access and manage network.

Reinhardt, U. E. (1995). Health reform is dead! Long live health reform! *Trends in Health Care, Law & Ethics, 10*(1–2), 7–10.

An examination of trends in the health care reform movement and on the nature of 21st-century American health care is presented. Capitated managed care will likely be the hallmark of future health care reform efforts.

Schauffler, H. H., & Rodriguez, T. (1993). Managed care for preventive services: A review of policy options. *Medical Care Review, 50*(2), 153–198.

In summary, the managed care system we propose for preventive services is designed to limit the potential for overcare under fee-for-service payment and for undercare under capitation and comprehensive fixed fees. It bases payment on the provision of a complete set of preventive services, thus limiting the tendency of physicians to provide only the relatively high-profit services, such as screening tests, while neglecting the lower-cost providers, such as laboratories, health educators and counselors, and community-based health promotion programs, thus encouraging greater efficiency. In addition, the proposed system funds both primary and high-risk factors. Finally, the proposed system monitors the use of preventive services, relying on physician reminders to stimulate the appropriate provision of preventive care and denying payment for unauthorized care. Existing research suggests that none of the individual strategies for managed care can be expected to achieve all of the goals of managing and promoting the appropriate use of preventive services as defined by the U.S. Preventive Services Task Force (1989). To be most effective, we conclude that

144

the strategies need to be coordinated and integrated into the current health care delivery practices of health maintenance organizations, preferred provider organizations, and point-of-service plans.

2.2 Employer Perspective

Garnick, D. W., Hendricks, A. M., Dulski, J. D., Thorpe, K. E., & Horgan, C. (1994). Characteristics of private-sector managed care for mental health and substance abuse treatment. *Hospital Community Psychiatry, 45*(12), 1201–1205.

This study examined diversity during the late 1980s in managed care programs for mental health, alcohol abuse, and drug abuse to identify ways in which research can generate more meaningful data on the effectiveness of utilization review programs. Methods: Telephone interviews were conducted with representatives of utilization review programs for employee health insurance plans in 31 firms that employed 2.1 million people in 1990. Results: Large variations in utilization review programs were found. Programs employed a range of review personnel and used a variety of clinical criteria to authorize care. More than two-thirds did not carve out mental health and substance abuse review from medical-surgical review. Conclusions: Because of trends toward even more diversity in utilization review programs in the 1990s, research that identifies the specific features of managed care programs that hold most promise for controlling costs while maintaining quality of care will increasingly be needed.

Moskowitz, D. B. (1995). Perspectives. Big payers, HMOs unite around quality measurement system. *Faulkner Grays Medical Health, 49*(19), suppl. 1–4.

Niemeyer, L. O., Foto, M., & Holmes-Enix, D. (1994). Perspectives: Implementing managed care in an industrial rehabilitation program. *Work: A Journal of Prevention, Assessment & Rehabilitation, 4*(1), 2–8.

Managed care, with all its problems and potentials, is entering the scene in workers' compensation as a way to deal with escalating costs. Though the roots of managed care lie in cost containment efforts, its future depends on a shift in emphasis to quality of care. Clinicians must become partners with insurance companies and employers to evolve a "win-win" scenario that combines efficiency with effectiveness or risk both exclusion from provider networks and loss of control over what becomes incorporated into standards of care. Steps that can be taken by clinicians include developing a sense of accountability for final functional outcomes, internal utilization management, and an internal case management protocol.

Potter, R. L. (1995). An integrated ethics program for managed care organizations. *Trends in Health Care, Law & Ethics, 10*(1–2), 87–90.

An integrated ethics program for managed care organizations is described. The object of this program is to create an ethical corporate culture in the health care environment.

Reiff, M. G., & Sperling, K. L. (1995). Measuring the savings from managed care: Experience at Citibank. *Benefits Quarterly, 11*(2), 19–25.

Scroggins, E. S. (1994). Employer demands lower cost. *Managed Care Quarterly, 2*(1), 72–76, discussion 87–88.

A case study of premium negotiations between a health maintenance organization (HMO) and an employer group is presented. The employer HMO and employer had a well-established relationship for several years. In the fourth year of consecutive double-digit rate increases, the employer demanded a decrease in premiums. The ensuing negotiations included the employer's mandate that the HMO make operational changes to effect cost reductions. The HMO was able to provide sufficient evidence supporting its position in the rate increase and subsequently a premium increase of 5 percent was negotiated. The case study is followed in subsequent articles by the opinions and commentary of executives in the managed care industry.

Slomski, A. J. (1994). How business is flattening health costs. *Medical Economist, 71*(13), 86–90, 92–93, 96 passim.

3. Reimbursement/Funding

Smith, B. C., & Elberth, W. (1993). Expanding payment: Managed care: The key to reimbursement in mental health. *OT Week, 7*(14), 22–23.

Weissenstein, E. (1995). Treat providers like insurers—NAIC. *Modern Healthcare, 25*(34), 24.

3.1 Medicare

Beebe, J. C. (1992). An outlier pool for Medicare HMO payments. *Health Care Financial Review, 14*(1), 59–63.

Medicare pays at-risk health maintenance organizations a prospective capitation amount that is established by the adjusted average per capita cost (AAPCC) formula for estimating the amount enrollees would have cost had they remained in the fee-for-service sector. Because the AAPCC accounts for a very small percentage of the variation in beneficiary costs, considerable research has been devoted to improving the formula. This article examines one approach to a payment system that combines the AAPCC with an outlier payment mechanism.

Schauffler, H. H., Howland, J., & Cobb, J. (1992). Using chronic disease risk factors to adjust Medicare capitation payments. *Health Care Financial Review, 14*(1), 79–90.

This study evaluates the use of risk factors for chronic disease as health status adjusters for Medicare's capitation formula, the average adjusted per capita costs (AAPCC). Risk factor data for the surviving members of the Framingham Study cohort who were examined in 1982–83 were merged with 100 percent Medicare payment data for 1984 and 1985, matching on Social Security number and sex. Seven different AAPCC models were estimated to assess the independent contributions of risk factors and measures of prior utilization and disability in increasing the explanatory power of AAPCC. The findings suggest that inclusion of risk factors for chronic disease as health status adjusters can improve substantially the predictive accuracy of AAPCC.

Weisblatt, M. (1995). What OTs should know about Medicare managed care. *OT Week, 9*(21), 20–22.

With more and more Medicare beneficiaries expected to join managed care plans in the future, it is essential that occupational therapy practitioners know how their services are covered.

3.2 Medicaid

Barry, P., & Schafer, A. (1993). Economics of a rehabilitation program for patients with a traumatic brain injury requiring long-term care. *The Journal of Head Trauma Rehabilitation, 8*(4), 48–58.

Arizona's public health care demonstration project, a managed care alternative to Medicaid, provides the context for a system with an incentive to contain costs. Within this context, a countywide network of rehabilitation programs has been developed to encourage placement and support of severely disabled people in the community, thereby reducing the need for long-term nursing home placements. This article describes the statewide system and the local rehabilitation network. Results of its first few years of operation suggest that coordinated rehabilitation programming is consistent with managed care objectives in long-term care and contributes to cost-effectiveness.

Bergen, S. S., Jr. (1995). Medicaid managed care. *Trends in Health Care, Law & Ethics, 10*(1–2), 132.

Factors that have motivated states to restructure Medicaid programs along a managed care model are discussed. Efforts are being made to integrate Medicaid recipients into the mainstream of health care delivery.

Freund, D. A., & Hurley, R. E. (1995). Medicaid managed care: Contribution to issues of health reform. *Annual Review of Public Health, 16*, 473–495.

This chapter examines the emergence of managed care in Medicaid from an alternative to the mainstream delivery system for many beneficiaries. It offers a definition that encompasses the broad spectrum of program manifestations and presents a brief historical perspective on the major eras of managed care in Medicaid. The major program prototypes are described and their contribution to enrollment growth is discussed. Research evidence is examined to address both operational issues and program impacts. Finally, we conclude with an appraisal of contemporary issues of importance and speculation on the next generation of Medicaid managed care programs with an eye toward how federal and state health care reform proposals will shape this future.

Monack, D. R. (1995). Medicaid and managed care: Opportunities for innovative service delivery to vulnerable populations. *Behavioral Healthcare Tomorrow, 4*(2), 19–23.

Ortolon, K. (1994). Taming the Medicaid beast. Lawmakers are looking to managed care to rein in escalating costs. *Texas Medicine, 90*(8), 32–35.

Pallak, M. S., Cummings, N. A., Dorken, H., & Henke, C. J. (1994). Medical costs, Medicaid, and managed mental health treatment: The Hawaii study. *Managed Care Quarterly, 2*(2), 64–70.

In a randomized, prospective design with Medicaid enrollees, managed mental health treatment reduced medical services costs and use by 23 to 40 percent relative to control groups. For enrollees with chronic medical diagnoses, managed treatment reduced medical costs by 28 to 47 percent, while medical costs for fee for service also reduced medical costs by about 20 percent but used three times as many outpatient visits. Costs of managed treatment were recovered in 6 to 24 months, suggesting that managed mental health treatment should be incorporated in health reform initiatives.

Sherman, S. J. (1995). Medicaid managed care keys to success. *Medical Group Management Journal, 42*(2), 12.

3.3 Private Insurance

Kertesz, L. (1995). Blues forms national network for managed-care Medicare. *Modern Healthcare, 25*(32), 18.

3.4 Workers' Compensation

Niemeyer, L. O., & Foto, M. (1994). Managed care: Partnering in workers' compensation. *REHAB Management, 7*(4), 138–141.

A philosophical shift toward active cooperation among providers, insurers, and employers is improving the efficiency of the workers' compensation system.

Niemeyer, L. O., & Foto, M. (1994). Managed care: The worker's comp dilemma. *REHAB Management, 7*(2), 109–111, 115.

The evolution of managed care in industrial rehab has so far made little allowance for the complex circumstances impacting injured workers.

3.5 Other Funding

Carter, A. M., & van Vleet, M. A. (1995). CHAMPUS psychiatric inpatient savings: Military management versus contractor, the Fort Polk experience. *Military Medicine, 160*(5), 242–247.

Jones, K. R. (1995). The changing reimbursement environment. *Seminars in Nursing Management, 3*(1), 5–6.

3.6 Marketing

Cohn, R. (1994). Strategies for positioning in the managed health care marketplace. *Journal of Hand Therapy, 7*(1), 5–9.

This articles defines managed health care, illustrated its continued growth, demonstrates its effect on clinical decision-making and reimbursement issues, and suggests strategies for optimal positioning in the managed care marketplace. The hand therapy specialist—whether based in a hospital, an institutional-based ambulatory care setting, or a private practice—must be aware of a managed plan's contractual limitations. Parameters discussed are patient length of stay, documentation, reimbursement, patient responsibility, alternatives to conventional treatment protocols, and the potential effects of utilization review on patient treatment. A provider must be well prepared to ensure delivery of quality care within the myriad restrictions imposed by managed care regulations.

Joe, B. E. (1994). Hand therapy: Preventing future shock under managed care. *OT Week, 8*(10), 18–19.

3.7 Documentation

Byrne, S. B. (1995). Getting real about capitation. *Hospital Health Network, 69*(17), 66.

Mangiante, L. (1995). A checklist for contracts. *Hospital Practitioner, 30*(3), 45–46.

Windle, P. E. (1994). Critical pathways: An integrated documentation tool. *Nursing Management, 25*(9), 80F–80L, 80P.

A multipurpose six-page, threefold flow sheet improves patient outcomes, meets JCAHO standards, and facilitates easy tracking of a patient's progress. The flow sheet is divided into nursing process, expected patient outcomes, critical pathway, and variance report. Outcomes management is an effective process to control costs and improve patient outcomes.

3.8 Capitation

Coile, R. C., Jr. (1994). Eight strategies for capitation. *Hospital Strategy Representative, 6*(12), 4–8.

Coile, R. C., Jr. (1994). The five stages of managed care. Organizing for capitation and health reform. *Hospital Strategy Representative, 6*(11), 1, 3, 8.

Friedman, B. B. (1995). Material executives and the managed cost continuum in a capitated environment. *Hospital Material Management Quarterly, 17*(1), 1–6.

Kolb, D. S., & Horowitz, J. L. (1995). Managing the transition to capitation. *Healthcare Financial Management, 49*(2), 64–69.

Although most experts believe that capitation and financial risk sharing among providers will become key components of the U.S. health care system, providers may not feel the full effect of this shift for several years. In the interim, providers must operate under an activity-based payment system that rewards them for the volume of patients seen, while preparing for the transition to a fixed, per capita payment system that will reward them for the efficiency with which services are provided. Preparation for the move to capitation will involve implementation of the systems necessary to negotiate managed care contracts, enhance quality and efficiency, and take responsibility for the health of a defined population.

Manton, K. G., Newcomer, R., Vertrees, J. C., Lowrimore, G. R., & Harrington, C. (1994). A method for adjusting capitation payments to managed care plans using multivariate patterns of health and functioning: The experience of social/health maintenance organizations.

A multivariate procedure for identifying case-mix dimensions from discrete health variables is presented. Since the dimensions are generated only from health use data and not service use data, they can be used for adjusted capitation rates to provide incentives to treat persons not currently well integrated into standard health care system (e.g., the very ill, the uninsured) or to promote specific health outcomes. The procedure is illustrated with data from social/health maintenance organizations (S/HMO) since they provide both acute and long-term care services. Thus, case-mix measures to adjust S/HMO reimbursements have to represent both medical conditions and the degree, and type, of functional impairment. From 31 health and functioning items, six case-mix dimensions, and scores for individuals on each, were calculated. The multivariate distribution of scores in S/HMO enrollees, and in Medicare-eligible comparison samples, were examined in each site to see how their health differed. S/HMO enrollees were healthier and less frail than people remaining in the Medicare fee-for-service system. Such differences are important in adjusting capitation rates to provide incentive to accept clients with complex health problems.

Newhouse, J. P., Sloss, E. M., Manning, W. G., Jr., & Keeler, E. B. (1993). Risk adjustment for a children's capitation rate. *Health Care Financial Review, 15*(1), 39–54.

Few capitation arrangements vary premiums by a child's health characteristics, yielding an incentive to discriminate against children with predictably high expenditures from chronic diseases. In this article, we explore risk adjusters for the 35 percent of the variance in annual outpatient expenditure we find to be potentially predictable. Demographic factors such as age and gender only explain 5 percent of such variance; health status measures explain 25 percent, prior use and health status measures together explain 65 to 70 percent. The profit from risk selection falls less than proportionately with improved ability to adjust for risk. Partial capitation rates may be necessary to mitigate skimming and dumping.

Ruffin, M. (1995). Capitation and informatics. *Physician Executives, 21*(7), 21–25.

When physicians, hospitals, and allied health professionals bill for services they render, their information processing requirements are relatively simple, at least compared with those of capitated organizations. When payers (insurers or employers) accept financial risk for the health care services of beneficiaries, they have usually invested in claims processing, membership tracking, and, under managed care, utilization review and provider profiling systems. In this article, we will explore why informatics is so important to capitated organizations and why payers that have traditionally taken financial risk for insuring the health care costs of populations are also learning about the importance of informatics.

3.9 Contracting Alliances

Caesar, N. B. (1994). Don't get burned by the boilerplate in your managed care contract. *Managed Care, 3*(2), 53–54.

Caesar, N. B. (1994). Two more snares to beware in contract boilerplate. *Managed Care, 3*(3), 51.

Clark, B. W. (1995). Negotiating successful managed care contracts. *Healthcare Financial Management, 49*(8), 26–30.

The goal in managed care contracting is to create a coherent framework for treatment and payment decisions that is as unintrusive, flexible, and cooperative as possible for both payers and providers. The goal is rarely achieved with a generic contract that ignores the circumstances and interests unique to a particular payer and provider. This article highlights a number of key issues that arise in managed care contracting in general and offers several practical suggestions for resolving those issues.

Goodrow, J. H., & Murphy, D. A. (1994). The algebra of managed care. Creating physician and hospital partnerships. *Hospital Topics, 72*(4), 14–18.

Lane, W. (1994). What the contract doesn't say. *Managed Care, 3*(4), 40, 42.

Moran, G. F. (1993). Rate structuring in managed care contracts demands detailed information. *Medical Group Management Journal, 40*(4), 9–10, 13.

In summary, managed care contracts are being written in a variety of ways, versions of capitation and discounted fee for service being only two of them. If you can't generate all of the information needed to negotiate, you need to step back and take another look at your management information system. Managed care is here. It was just around the corner yesterday!

Mowery, N. R. (1994). The 10 most important clauses in a managed care contract. *Indiana Medicine, 87*(4), 284–287.

Robbins, K. S. (1995). Legal liability under managed care. *Hawaii Medical Journal, 54*(4), 490–494.

> Market forces are driving the delivery of health care into managed care. New alignments among health care providers, payers, utilization reviewers, and hospitals create new legal liability. Better-informed patients, concurrent credentialing by hospitals and payers, and new incentives to reduce hospital and physician-related costs have resulted in new federal legislation and agencies that reshape health care delivery and legal liability.

20 questions every physician should ask about managed-care contracts. (1994). *Postgraduate Medicine, 95*(3), 59–60, 63.

3.10 General

Barry, P., & Schafer, A. (1993). Economics of a rehabilitation program for patients with a traumatic brain injury requiring long-term care. *The Journal of Head Trauma Rehabilitation, 8*(4), 48–58.

> Arizona's public health care demonstration project, a managed care alternative to Medicaid, provides the context for a system with an incentive to contain costs. Within this context, a countrywide network of rehabilitation programs has been developed to encourage placement and support of severely disabled people in the community, thereby reducing the need for long-term nursing home placements. This article describes the statewide system and the local rehabilitation network. Results of its first few years of operation suggest that coordinated rehabilitation programming is consistent with managed care objectives in long-term care and contributes to cost-effectiveness.

Cohn, R. (1994). Strategies for positioning in the managed health care marketplace. *Journal of Hand Therapy, 7*(1), 5–9.

> This article defines managed health care, illustrates its continued growth, demonstrates its effect on clinical decision-making and reimbursement issues, and suggests strategies for optimal positioning in the managed care marketplace. The hand therapy specialist—whether based in a hospital, an institution-based ambulatory care setting, or a private practice—must be aware of a managed plan's contractual limitations. Parameters discussed are patient length of stay, documentation, reimbursement, patient responsibility, alternatives to conventional treatment protocols, and the potential effects of utilization review on patient treatment.

Kertesz, L. (1994). Efficiencies help curb HMO rates. *Modern Healthcare, 24*(47), 82.

Kranther, M. A. (1994). The gatekeeper in managed care. *Journal of Healthcare Risk Management, 14*(4), 8–10.

Murcko, A. C. (1995). Managed care: Winning (and losing) in the West. *Internist, 36*(5), 6–7.

4. Management

Hoffman, E., & Johnson, K. (1995). Women's health and managed care: Implications for the training of primary care physicians. *Journal of American Womens Association, 50*(1), 17-19.

Wartman, S. A. (1994). Managed care and its effect on residency training in internal medicine. *Archives of Internal Medicine, 154*(22), 2539-2544.

Weitekamp, M. R., & Ziegenfuss, J. T. (1995). Academic health centers and HMOs: A system perspective on collaboration in training generalists physicians and advancing mutual interests. *Academic Medicine, 70*(1 Suppl.), S47-S53.

4.1 Outcomes

Bailit, H., Federico, J., & McGivney, W. (1995). Use of outcomes studies by a managed care organization: Valuing measured treatment effects. Aetna Health plans. *Medicare Care, 33*(4 Suppl.), AS216-225.

Burlingame, G. M., Lambert, M. J., Reisinger, C. W., Neff, W. M., & Mosier, J. (1995). Pragmatics of tracking mental health outcomes in a managed care setting. *Journal of Mental Health Administration, 22*(3), 226-236.

Mayhan, Y. D. (1994). The importance of outcomes measurement in managed care. *Administration & Management Special Interest Section Newsletter, 10*(4), 2-4.

Nugent, W. C., & Schults, W. C. (1994). Playing by the numbers: How collecting outcomes data changed my life. *Annals of Thoracic Surgery, 58*(6), 1866-1870.

The Northern New England Cardiovascular Study Group has been using clinical epidemiology to analyze outcomes data in patients undergoing cardiac surgical procedures to answer three questions: (1) for the surgeon: How am I doing? (2) for the patient: What are my chances? and (3) for society: Can outcomes data be voluntarily collected and organized in a way to improve care delivery? The Dartmouth-Hitchcock Medical Center cardiac surgery program has combined these regional outcomes data with the internal development of critical pathways; with evaluations of patient expectations, patient satisfaction, and patient functional health; and with innovative techniques of data display in an effort to improve the cardiac surgical outcomes in patients at the center. The length of stay has declined, and both the mortality rate and readmission rate have remained stable.

Odderson, I. R., & McKenna, B. S. (1993). A model for management of patients with stroke during the acute phase. Outcome and economic implications. *Stroke, 24*(12), 1823-1827.

The purpose of the study was to develop a clinical pathway for patients with non-hemorrhagic stroke during the acute hospital phase to improve the quality of care and reduce costs. The pathway included standard admission orders and a swallow screen on Day 1 of hospitalization. Physical therapy, occupational therapy, speech therapy, and social worker assessments were done on Day 2. A physiatry consult was performed on Day 3 if indicated, and by Day 4 a discharge target date and disposition were addressed. Outcomes for 121 patients during the first year of pathway implementation are reported. Average length of stay on the acute service decreased from 10.9 days to 7.3 days (P<.05), reducing the charges per patient by 14.6 percent. Complications in the form of urinary tract infections and aspiration pneumonia rates decreased by 63.2 percent (P<.05) and 38.7 percent, respectively. We conclude that the implementation of a clinical pathway for patients with acute, nonhemorrhagic stroke resulted in a significant reduction in length of stay, charges, and complications while improving the quality of care.

Pace, K. B. (1995). Data sets for home care organizations. *Caring, 14*(3), 38–42.

Tapper, B. E. (1994). ASHT launches outcomes data collection system. *OT Week, 8*(50), 20–21.

> With moves toward managed care, outcomes data are becoming increasingly important. A new computerized data collection system may help therapists enter this new arena.

Woodyard, L. W., & Sheetz, J. E. (1993). Critical pathway patient outcomes: The missing standard. *Journal of Nursing Care Quality, 8*(1), 51–57.

4.2 Case Management

Collier, P., & Early, A. (1995). A team approach to geriatric case management. *Journal of Case Management, 4*(2), 66–70.

Guinan, J. K. (1993). Facility-based case management: Its role in rehabilitation nursing. *Rehabilitation Nursing, 18*(4), 254–256, 261.

Hinzman, C. (1994). Case management experience helps RN students incorporate professional role attributes. *Nursing Education, 19*(4), 6.

Joe, B. E. (1995). Case managers confront managed care. *OT Week, 9*(41), 14–15.

> Case managers who once saw themselves primarily as client advocates are now balancing client care against the viability of their facility.

Nelson, M. M. (1993). The race for victory in rehabilitation case management. *Rehabilitation Nursing, 18*(4), 253–254.

Price, J. (1993). The impact of case management on psychiatry. *NAHAM Management Journal, 18*(3), 10–11.

Zander, K. (Ed.). (1991). CareMaps™: The core of cost/quality care. *The New Definition, 6*(3), 2-4.

Zander, K. (Ed.). (1992). Physicians, CareMaps™, and collaboration. *The New Definition, 7*(1), 1-3.

Zander, K. (Ed.). (1992). Quantifying, managing, and improving quality, part I: How caremaps™ link CQI to the patient. *The New Definition, 7*(1), 1–3.

Zander, K. (Ed.). (1992). Quantifying, managing, and improving quality, part II: The collaborative management of quality care. *The New Definition, 7*(3), 1–2.

Zander, K. (Ed.). (1992). Quantifying, managing, and improving quality, part III: Using variance concurrently. *The New Definition, 7*(4), 1–3.

4.3 Utilization Review/Quality Assurance/Risk Management

Chester, J., Sanguineti, V. R., Samuel, S. E., Dichter, H., & Glacken, M. (1995). Providers and reviewers teach informed managed care. *Medical Interface, 8*(5), 124–126.

> Two utilization review case studies are summarized, with discussion of both the provider's and the reviewer's perspective. This interface between managed care organizations and behavioral health care professionals offers some instructive guidelines on how to best approach that utilization review process.

Foto, M., & Swanson, G. (1993). Utilization review & managed care. *REHAB Management, 6*(5), 123–125.

> Continued growth in managed care and cost-containment initiative means increased use of UR, with important practice implications.

Furrow, B. R. (1995). Managed care and the evolution of quality. *Trends in Health Care, Law & Ethics, 10*(1–2), 37–44.

> The impact that managed care plans are having on the evolution of quality health care in the United States is assessed. Managed care plans impose financial disincentives for doctors to treat, refer, or hospitalize patients.

Goldfield, N. (1994). Case mix, risk adjustment, reinsurance, and health reform. *Management Care Quarterly, 2*(3), iv–viii.

> Case-mix measures represent the fundamental tool used to ascertain clinical differences in groups of patients. It is important to use these measures carefully, as quality of care delivered to patients is at stake. Risk adjustment methodologies are excellent for physician profiling if one adopts them as the first step in the quality improvement process. Differences in hospital or primary care practice profiles, adjusted for the case-mix measures, often reveal quality improvement opportunities. This first step is easy. The hard part comes in working together with the health care team to determine the sources for these differences. In turn, this will provide the health care team with a greater ability to deal with treasures uncovered by applying case-mix measures.

Guerette, P. H. (1995). Managed care: Cookbook medicine, or quality, cost-effective care? *Canadian Nursing, 91*(7), 16.

Harding J. (1994). Risk management in an IPA setting—Part I. *Physician Executive, 20*(5), 32–37.

> Over the past several years, health maintenance organization (HMO) enrollment has grown the most in independent practice association (IPA) and network models. HMOs in general have expanded as a means to control the cost of health care. IPA and the network models retain a greater sense of choice on the part of participating physicians and patients than do closed-panel group- or staff-model programs. This two-part article examines the differences between staff-model and IPA-model HMOs in liability and in ability to manage risk. In the first part, the nature of the risks is described. In the next issue of the journal, the management of those risks is discussed.

Hersch, R. G. (1994). Mental health's contribution to the financial performance of a utilization management program. *Managed Care Quarterly, 2*(2), 64–70.

Analysis of a national utilization management program covering approximately 3.4 million individuals from 1989 through June 1993 indicates that while only 6 percent of all hospitalizations were for a primary psychiatric or substance abuse diagnosis, over 44 percent of the program savings are accounted for by concurrent mental health utilization management. The cost of performing mental health utilization management is significantly greater than the cost of providing medical, surgical, and maternity management, but returns on investments are significantly greater for psychiatric and substance abuse than for these other diagnostic areas. Implications for health care reform inclusion of full mental health benefits are discussed.

Kelly, J. T., & Kelly, J. M. (1995). Evaluating quality of care in fee-for-service and managed care delivery systems: Recommendations for quality leaders. *Quality Letters of Healthcare Leaders, 7*(3), 10–14.

Lazarus, A. (1994). Using an appeals panel to mediate mental health care UR disputes. *Medical Interface, 7*(8), 56–58, 76.

The certification of admission and lengthy psychiatric hospitalizations raise fundamental issues related to the appropriateness of treatment. The author presents several case examples to illustrate how an appeals panel resolves disputed utilization review decisions regarding inpatient psychiatric treatment.

Lazarus, A. (1995). Relational triangles in managed care. *Medical Interface, 8*(8), 71–72, 74.

Relational triangles provide a conceptual framework for understanding interpersonal relationships and utilization review disputes in managed care programs. Relational triangles exist in the everyday practice of medicine. The most striking example of relational triangles in practice is found in managed care systems' concurrent utilization management programs. The author provides some rules of relational triangles and vignettes to illustrate how they work in the managed care setting.

Pine, M., & Harper, D. L. (1994). Designing and using case mix indices. *Managed Care Quarterly, 2*(3), 1–11.

Quick, B. (1994). Integrating case management and utilization management. *Nurse Management, 25*(11), 52–56.

Over the years, the utilization review coordinator's role has evolved to more than quality assessment, risk management, and utilization management. Recognizing the need to expand the traditional role, one hospital integrated two positions: case management and utilization management. A two-month pilot study defining roles, responsibilities, outcomes, and future goals is described.

Ray, J. (1995). The marriage of risk management and the processes of patient care. *Physician Executives, 21*(7), 9–14.

Schoenbaum, S. C. (1993). Using evidence for utilization management: An HMO manager's perspective. *Annals of New York Academy of Science, 703*, 272–274.

Schwarz, T. (1994). Continuous quality improvement and the utilization management process. *Medical Interface, 7*(8), 77–78, 83–85, 101.

How does a managed health plan create a formalized utilization management program using quality improvement processes? One HMO is going through this process, trying to keep a Byzantine project simple through Deming's teachings. The author recounts this managed care organization's experiences.

Sennett, C., Legorreta, A. P., & Zatz, S. L. (1993). Performance-based hospital contracting for quality improvement. *Joint Commission Journal of Quality Improvement, 19*(9), 374–383.

Wells, K. B., Astrachan, B. M., Tischler, G. L., & Unutzer, J. (1995). Issues and approaches in evaluating managed mental health care. *Milbank Quarterly, 73*(1), 57–75.

Data on the ways in which alternative forms of managed care affect the costs, quality, and outcomes of mental health are needed to inform health policy and clinical care decisions. Such evaluations, however, are difficult to implement for conceptual and practical reasons. The definition of managed mental health care is reviewed, alternative forms are described, and the activities and procedures that constitute managed care are identified.

Zablocki, E. (1994). Strategies for ensuring access and appropriate utilization under managed care. *Quality Lett Healthcare Leaders, 6*(2), 2–11.

4.4 Workforce Supervision/Staffing

Daz'e, C. (1994). Patients can get data on doctors just by picking up the phone. *Managed Care, 3*(6), 53.

Frampton, J., & Wall, S. (1994). Exploring the use of NPs and PAs in primary care. *HMO Practice, 8*(4), 165–170.

Hettinger, J. (1995). Training competent aides. *OT Week, 9*(41), 18–19.

Spaulding Rehabilitation Hospital in Boston effective managed care calls for the creative use of staff members. Competently trained and supervised OT aides are helping COTAs and OTRs deliver quality care.

How do non-physician providers function in HMOs? (1994). *HMO Practice, 8*(4), 151–156.

Hummel, J., & Pirzada, S. (1994). Estimating the cost of using non-physician providers in primary care teams in an HMO: Where would the savings begin? *HMO Practice, 8*(4), 162–164.

Kelley, S. K., & Trautlein, J. J. (1992). A survey of human resources in managed care organizations. *Physician Executive, 18*(6), 49–51.

Although managed health care is increasing exponentially in the United States, minimal published information exists regarding the human resources needed to perform various managed care activities. This article reports on the results of a national survey of managed care organizations regarding the quantitative use of nurse and physician reviewers and the type of activities being performed.

Loveridge, C. E. (1995). Preparing the workforce for managed care. *Seminars in Nursing Management, 3*(2), 89–94.

Theirs, N. (1994). What will manage care mean for COTAs? *OT Week, 8*(11), 23.

Well, T. P., & Miller, W. H. (1995). Some implications of managed care for physician assistants. *Physician Assistant, 19*(2), 63–66, 69–70, 72–74.

4.5 Public Relations

Mangan, D. (1995). From ally to enemy. The ugly split between 175 doctors and Prudential. *Medical Economist, 72*(6), 26–28, 30–35, 39.

Miller, J. L. (1994). Role of physician extenders on the managed care team. *Integrated Healthcare Representative,* 8–11.

Nelson, A. R. (1994). Gatekeeper: Guide or guard? *Internist, 35*(4), 25.

Stahl, D. A. (1995). Managed care credentialing. *Nursing Management, 26*(6), 18–19.

Terry, P. E., & Pheley, A. (1993). The effect of self-care brochures on use of medical services. *Journal of Occupational Medicine, 35*(4), 422–426.

Zalta, E. (1994). Is success spelled g-a-t-e-k-e-e-p-e-r? *Medical Interface, 7*(4), 123–129.

4.6 Marketing/Cost Analysis

McAuley, L. T. (1993). Administrative and operational responsibilities in contract management. *Top Health Care Finance, 20*(2), 76–81.

Frequently, chief financial officers or marketing executives negotiate contracts that are difficult if not impossible to implement. In addition, those parties responsible for implementing contracts are often unaware of the terms. Formal verbal and written communications within a health care organization will minimize consumer (payer and patient) displeasure, as well as alleviate internal frustration and stress.

Thiers, N. (1994). Facing foreign territory: As managed care becomes more entranced in our health care system, OTs in private practice must adjust their business approach. *OT Week, 8*(33), 16–19.

4.7 Documentation

Indexing for inflation: A critical step in managed care calculations. *Hospital Cost Management Accounting, 6*(8), 4–6.

Parsi, K. P., Winslade, W. J., & Corcoran, K. (1995). Does confidentiality have a future? The computer-based patient record and managed mental health care. *Trends in Health Care, Law & Ethics, 10*(1–2), 78–82.

The impact of managed care on ethical and legal aspects of privacy/confidentiality in mental health care is examined. Greater safeguards governing the use of computer-based patient records must be established to protect patient privacy and confidentiality.

4.8 Critical/Clinical Pathways

American Medical Association. (1993). *Directory of practice parameters: Titles, sources, and updates.* Chicago: AMA Office of Quality Assurance and Medical Review.

Capuano, T. A. (1995). Clinical pathways: Practical approaches, positive outcomes. *Nursing Management, 26*(1), 34–37.

There is an obvious need to restructure delivery of health care, implementation of changes often takes place under less than ideal circumstances. Strategies are presented for implementing clinical pathways, with a focus on global, organizational issues encountered in the real world.

Dowling, W. J., Frommer, A. G., & O'Keefe, T. (1995). Critical pathways in total joint procedures. *Strategic Healthcare Excellence, 8*(3), 9–12.

Drazen, E. C., Metzger, J. B., & Stasior, D. S. (1994). Letter to the editor. *New England Journal of Medicine, 330,* 436.

Dunn, J., Rodriquez, D., & Novak, J. J. (1994). Promoting quality mental health care delivery with critical path care plans. *Journal of Psychosocial Nursing and Mental Health Services, 32*(7), 25–29.

Mental health providers are under increasing pressure to provide objective, individualized care that produces outcomes that may be measured against accepted clinical standards. Clinicians may now track patient responses throughout a continuum of treatment in varying locations by using a customized critical path/treatment plan format. Care delivery is documented by superimposing actual occurrences over desired ones on a critical pathway.

Farley, K. (1995). The COPD critical pathway: A case study in progress. *Quality Management Health Care, 3*(2), 43–54.

Patients with chronic obstructive pulmonary disease (COPD) consume many health care resources and require complex coordination of care among multiple caregivers. In this report, we share our experiences at Fletcher Allen Health Care, Burlington, Vermont, in developing and implementing a critical pathway for these patients. The COPD pathway has resulted in measurable improvements in the quality of care and has provided us with lessons that will enhance our use of critical pathway methods.

Frantz, A. (1994). The cardiac care step-down unit at home. *Caring, 13*(10), 42–48, 51.

Clinical pathways have proven to be the key to shortening hospital stays for cardiac patients, allowing them to move out of the hospital and return home sooner. These pathways have truly facilitated the paradigm shift from institutional to home care.

Geradi, T. (1994). A regional hospital association's approach to clinical pathway development. *Journal of Healthcare Quality, 16*(5), 10–14.

Sixteen hospitals from the Northeastern New York Hospital Council tested the theory that clinical pathways are an essential component of the integrated quality assessment process. Clinical pathways served as a transition to the holistic, process-oriented approach of quality improvement. The clinical pathways that they developed included preadmission, hospitalization, and postdischarge care needs. This regional approach to care resulted in increased patient and staff satisfaction, positive patient outcomes, and a decrease in length of stay.

Graham, M. J., Pettus, T., & Klava, S. (1995). Subacute care. Critical pathways link services to outcomes. *Provider, 21*(9), 31–32.

Greenfield, E. (1995). Critical pathways: What they are and what they are not. *Journal of Burn Care Rehabilitation, 16*(2, Pt. 2), 196–197.

Hydo, B. (1995). Designing an effective clinical pathway for stroke. *American Journal of Nursing, 95*(3), 44–50.

Jaklevic, M. C. (1995). Doc practice management set to explode. *Modern Healthcare, 25*(33), 26–28, 30–31.

Johnson, M. D, & Morrison, M. (1995). Service options under managed care: How to reap savings. *Journal of Healthcare Resource Management, 13*(8), 28, 31–32.

Korpiel, M. R. (1995). Issues related to clinical pathways: Managed care, implementation, and liability. *Journal of Burn Care Rehabilitation, 16*(2, Pt. 2), 191–195.

Martich, D. (1993). The role of the nurse educator in the development of critical pathways. *Journal of Nursing Staff Development, 9*(5), 227–229.

This article focuses on the role of the nurse educator in developing critical pathways. It serves as a guide for the nurse educator by defining how critical pathways support managed care, identifying the goals of critical pathway education, and reviewing the importance of organizational commitment to the critical pathways before their use. The nurse educator serves as instructor, facilitator, and consultant in critical pathway development.

Milne, C. T., & Pelletier, L. C. (1994). Enhancing staff skill. Developing critical pathways at a community hospital. *Journal of Nursing Staff Development, 10*(3), 160–162.

Clinical pathways are an essential tool in implementing case management. The authors describe how one institution developed and implemented critical pathways. The result was enhanced staff skill in physical assessment, patient/family teaching, and communication with physicians.

Nelson, M. (1993). Critical pathways in the emergency department. *Journal of Emergency Nursing, 19*(2), 110–114.

Nyberg, D., & Marschke, P. (1993). Critical pathways: Tools for continuous quality improvement. *Nursing Administration Quarterly, Spring,* 62–69.

O'Leary, D. S. (1993). The measurement mandate: Report card day is coming. *Journal on Quality Improvement, 19,* 487–497.

Rozell, B. R., & Newman, K. L. (1994). Extending a critical path for patients who are ventilator dependent: Nursing case management in the home setting. *Home Healthcare in Nursing, 12*(4), 21–25.

A case management model is prepared to extend nursing care of the patient who is ventilator dependent from the hospital to the home setting. The model focuses on decreasing the hospital length of stay and major critical pathway elements. Effective discharge planning is emphasized.

Schriefer, J. (1995). Managing critical pathway variances. *Quality Managing Health Care, 3*(2), 30–42.

Variance management is not clearly defined in the literature, and many institutions search for the best approach. We have implemented a number of different techniques for variance management at Fletcher Allen Health Care. Our success benefits both patients and providers.

Stahl, D. A. (1995). Critical pathways in subacute care. *Nursing Management, 26*(9), 16–18.

4.9 Information Systems

Abbott, J., Hronek, C., & Mirecki, J. K. (1995). The leap to automating clinical pathways. *Journal of Healthcare Resources Manager, 13*(6), 8–16.

> There are a mind-boggling number of approaches an organization can take to realize cost and quality goals. These range from case management and paper clinical pathway systems to work redesign and computerization. Often an organization's first step toward better care management is to implement some form of clinical pathway system.

Bazzoli, F. (1995). Demonstrating how automation can improve outcomes. *Health Data Management, 3*(6), 41–42, 46–47.

Cagney, T., & Woods, D. R. (1994). Clinical management information systems. *Behavioral Healthcare Tomorrow, 3*(1), 43–45.

Caper, P. (1995). Shifting to a new medical care paradigm. *Infocare,* 46, 48, 50.

Crow, M. R., Smith, H. L., McNamee, A. H., & Piland, N. F. (1994). Considerations in predicting mental health care use: Implications for managed care plans. *Journal of Mental Health Administration, 21*(1), 5–23.

> Managed care plans and other health care providers face a difficult task in predicting outpatient mental health services use. Existing research offers some guidance, but our knowledge of which factors influence use is confounded by methodological problems and sampling constraints. Consequently, available findings are insufficient for developing accurate predictions, which managed care plans need to formulate fiscally responsible service delivery contracts. This article review the primary data sources and research on ambulatory mental health services. On the basis of this review, the probability and intensity of outpatient visits are estimated. The implications for planning capitated mental health services are discussed.

Geraty, R. (1995). Managed care systems require sophisticated data interactions. *Behavioral Healthcare Tomorrow, 4*(1), 42–43, 46–47.

Kane, R. L., Bartlett, J., & Potthoff, S. (1994). Integrating an outcomes information system into managed care for substance abuse. *Behavioral Healthcare Tomorrow, 3*(3), 57–61.

Kane, R. L., Bartlett, J., & Potthoff, S. (1995). Building an empirically based outcomes information system for managed mental health care. *Psychiatry Service, 46*(5), 459–461.

Keegan, A. J. (1995). The need to integrate clinical and financial information. *Healthcare Financial Management, 47*(7), 36–38.

Trabin, T. (1994). How will computerization revolutionize managed care? *Managed Care Quarterly, 2*(2), 22–24.

> Computerization of behavioral health care information systems is revolutionizing how payers, managed care companies, and providers exchange information. In this article, an imaginary scenario is depicted of how patient data will be accessed and communicated to facilitate care management of behavioral health care services in the near future.

4.10 General Management

Hiatt, D., & Hargrave, G. E. (1995). The characteristics of highly effective therapists in managed behavioral provider networks. *Behavioral Healthcare Tomorrow, 4*(4), 19–22.

As managed behavioral health care plans experience increasing requirements to measure outcomes, create report cards, and adopt other quantifiable approaches to quality management, rating the effectiveness of behavioral health care providers is essential. The authors describe one aspect of their company's quality management program, which uses standardized assessments of client satisfaction, problem resolution, and appropriateness of care to identify highly effective therapists. This process has yielded useful results that indicate some of the characteristics of highly effective therapists in such areas as experience, gender, and personality type.

Theis, G. A., Geraty, R., Panzarino, P. J., Jr., & Bartlett, J. (1995). Toward the behavioral health report card. *Medical Interface, 8*(3), 80–82, 122.

In this article, the authors review current organized efforts, strategies, and partnerships involved in attempts to design a behavioral health care report card that offers a comprehensive approach to obtaining performance measurements in the field of psychiatry and chemical dependence treatment.

5. Legal/Ethical

Costello, M. M., & Murphy, K. M. (1995). Clinical guidelines: A defense in medical malpractice suits. *Physician Executive, 21*(8), 10–12.

Clinical pathways, or practice guidelines, have been gaining wider acceptance from physicians and hospitals seeking to constrain increasing operating costs for inpatient care. The authors believe that properly developed and agreed-upon guidelines can also be used in certain cases as appropriate standards of care in determining whether medical malpractice has occurred. Adherence to the guidelines could then be asserted by defendants as an affirmative defense in a medical malpractice suit.

Dowell, M. A. (1993). Avoiding HMO liability for utilization review. *Special Law Digest Health Care Law, 171,* 9–32.

In this article, the author describes the potential liability of health maintenance organizations (HMOs) for utilization review programs. The author analyzes several recent cases and offers practical ideas for preventing and defending suits brought against HMOs for utilization review decisions.

Fiesta, J. (1995). Managed care: Whose liability? *Nursing Management, 26*(2), 31–32.

Montague, J. (1995). Playing by the rules: MD groups and antitrust. *Hospital Health Network, 69*(6), 56–58.

Miller, W. J. (1993). Legal considerations in managed care contracting. *Top Health Care Finance, 20*(2), 17–25.

Managed health care systems are created primarily through contracting. Although contracts with managed care organizations, such as health maintenance organizations, are often presented to providers as nonnegotiable, this article discusses basic contract terms that are frequently negotiated by the parties, including key contract definitions, compensation, term and termination, and boilerplate provisions. The article also emphasizes the need for contracting parties to conduct precontracting due diligence and to comply with applicable antitrust laws in negotiating contracts with groups of independent providers.

Morreim, E. H. (1995). The ethics of incentives in managed care. *Trends in Health Care, Law & Ethics, 10*(1–2), 56–62.

Ethical considerations related to managed care organizations (MCOs) on both a policy level and a clinical level are examined. Ideally, under a sound MCO, physicians' incentives could be shifted to promote quality of care.

Moskowitz, D. B. (1993). New court rulings threaten managed care's restrictive hiring, contracting practices. *Journal of American Health Policy, 3*(5), 49–52.

Olsen, D. P. (1994). The ethical considerations of managed care in mental health treatment. *Journal of Psychosocial Nursing in Mental Health Services, 32*(3), 25–28.

5.1 Fraud and Abuse

Tamborlane, T. A. (1994). Prohibited practices and safe harbors—A legal quagmire. *Caring, 13*(5), 32–34, 36–37.

Judging by the number and scope of laws they enact, legislators seem convinced that all health care entities need strict supervision via limits and prohibitions. This means that every contract a home care agency enters into needs thorough review and evaluation for numerous things.

5.2 Patient/Provider Relationship

Lazarus, A. (1994). Using an appeals panel to mediate mental health care UR disputes. *Medical Interface, 7*(8), 56–58, 76.

The certification of admission and lengthy psychiatric hospitalizations raise fundamental issues related to the appropriateness of treatment. The author presents several case examples to illustrate how an appeals panel resolves disputed utilization review decisions regarding inpatient psychiatric treatment.

Macklin, R. (1995). The ethics of managed care. *Trends in Health Care, Law & Ethics, 10* (1–2), 63–66.

Reasons why managed care is a bad omen for the doctor-patient relationship are discussed. Managed care contains some ethically questionable features that will undercut the already delicate doctor-patient relationship and compromise health care quality.

Mulholland, D. M., III. (1993). Managed care liability for medical malpractice and utilization review. *Medical Staff Counsel, 7*(2), 35–43.

Managed care subscribers alleging harm due to physician negligence often assert claims against their managed care plans as well. This article reviews five theories of liability under which relief has been sought and describes some of the defenses managed care organizations have raised to avoid liability.

Orentlicher, D. (1995). Managed care and the threat to the patient-physician relationship. *Trends in Health Care, Law & Ethics, 10*(1–2), 19–24.

Ways in which managed care threatens to undermine the patient-physician relationship are considered. Managed care plans have the potential to minimize the extent to which the physician's duty of loyalty to the patient is compromised.

Robbins, K. S. (1995). Legal liability under managed care. *Hawaii Medical Journal, 54*(4), 490–494.

Market forces are driving the delivery of health care into managed care. New alignments among health care providers, payers, utilization reviewers and hospitals create new legal liability. Better-informed patients, concurrent credentialing by hospitals and payers, and new incentives to reduce hospital and physician-related costs have resulted in new federal legislation and agencies that reshape health care delivery and legal liability.

Yarmolinsky, A. (1995). Sounding board: Supporting the patient. *New England Journal of Medicine, 332*(9), 602–603.

People who join health maintenance organizations put their health in the hands of primary care physicians who serve as gatekeepers to specialists. The independence of physicians is being impaired by business-owned managed-care companies, which may put a higher value on the bottom line than on the welfare of patients.

5.3 General Ethical/Legal Issues

AMA's ethics council is seeking physician comments (1995). *American Medical News, 38*(8), 20.

163

The AMA's Council on Ethical and Judicial Affairs is seeking comments from physicians for use in developing or revising five ethical reports on several topics, including managed care and prescription drug use.

Aroskar, M. A. (1995). Managed care and nursing values: A reflection. *Trends in Health Care, Law & Ethics, 10*(1–2), 83–86.

Beryy, K. (1995). Legislative forum: Maryland HEDIS report card project. *Journal of Healthcare Quality, 17*(5), 32.

Burns, E. (1994). Understanding liability issues in managed care. *QRC Advisory, 10*(5), 8–10.

Jecker, N. S. (1995). Business ethics and the ethics of managed care. *Trends in Health Care, Law & Ethics, 10*(1–2), 53–55.

Competing views about the ethical responsibilities of for-profit managed care plans and how managed care can be fashioned.

LaPuma, J., Schiedermayer, D., & Seigler, M. (1995). Ethical issues in managed care. *Trends in Health Care, Law & Ethics, 10*(1–2), 73–77.

Marren, J. P., & Hynes, D. W. (1995). Legal issues in accepting capitation. *Physician Executives, 21*(7), 15–20.

The effort to reduce the cost of medical, hospital, and ancillary services increasingly focuses on shifting the financial risk for the cost of these services to those who provide them. Shifting arrangements include capitation for physicians classified as primary care physicians; capitation arrangements that include primary and specialty services; risk shifting to medical groups, independent practice associations, and other physician organizations; and the packaging of physician and hospital services on a full-risk, per-case, or other basis. Accepting financial risk for the cost of medical and other health care services, as well as the responsibility for managing the provision of services, may very well be the only remaining opportunity for providers to maximize reimbursement and maintain administrative and clinical self-direction.

Moore, G. T., Inui, T. S., Ludden, J. M., Schoenbaum, S. C. (1994). The "teaching HMO": A new academic partner. *Academic Medicine, 69*(8), 595–600.

Potter, R. L. (1995). An integrated ethics program for managed care organizations. *Trends in Health Care, Law & Ethics, 10*(1–2), 87–90.

Purtilo, R. B. (1995). Managed care: Ethical issues for the rehabilitation professions. *Trends in Health Care, Law & Ethics, 10*(1–2), 105–108.

Ways in which medical ethics could be compromised by unintended consequences of managed care arrangements are examined, focusing on the rehabilitation professions. The outcomes approach to setting priorities and determining the parameters of quality care is emphasized.

Scofield, G. R. (1995). Mangled care. *Trends in Health Care, Law & Ethics, 10*(1–2), 47–52.

Flaws inherent in the managed care approach to health care reform are examined. Managed care would further legitimize a health care system that benefits health care providers rather than the patients they serve.

Tamborlane, T. (1995). Risk management: Navigating the legal waters of physician referral. *Trends in Health Care, Law & Ethics, 10*(1–2), 138–140.

In its OBRA laws and safe harbors, the federal government seeks to prohibit direct or indirect remuneration of physicians for patient referrals. Physicians must become familiar with the laws and regulations and use that knowledge to guide practice structure, referrals, and investments. Practices must comply with the regulations' intent; activities designed to meet safe harbors but which still generate illegal remuneration are not protected. Legal counsel can help physicians determine whether state or licensing agency requirements vary from federal requirements.

Thomasma, D. C. (1995). The ethics of managed care and cost control. *Trends in Health Care, Law & Ethics, 10*(1–2), 33–36.

The nature of managed care and the ethical challenges of cost cutting in the managed care environment are examined. A quality of life analysis would do much to individualize and personalize health care and limit unnecessary care.

6. Education

AMA-RPS priorities for 1995–1996. (1995). *Journal of the American Medical Association, 273*(23), 18060.

Physician workforce distribution and graduate medical education and funding, definition of economic hardship for loan deferment, resident work environment and managed care practice limitations were the areas that the AMA-RPS Governing Council indicated it would concentrate on for 1995–1996. These issues were addressed at the 1995 AMA annual meeting.

Carter, J. H. (1994). Provider and subscriber education: The key to survival. *Managed Care Quarterly, 2*(1), 83–84.

Charney, E. (1995). The education of pediatricians for primary care: The score after two score years. *Pediatrics, 95*(2), 270–272.

The extent to which pediatrics has addressed the issue of primary care education over the past two decades is discussed. There are clear indicators of pediatrics' commitment to generalism in practice and ongoing efforts to translate that commitment to the graduate education curriculum.

Church, G. J. (1995). Teaching hospitals in crisis. *Time, 146*(3), 40–42.

The teaching hospitals that train doctors and pioneer new procedures are scrambling to survive managed care and cutbacks. The survival of teaching hospitals, such as the UCLA Medical Center, is discussed.

Cohen, J. J. (1995). Educational mandates from managed care. *Academy of Medicine, 70*(5), 381.

Copeland, E. M., III, Flynn, T. C., & Ross, W. E. (1995). Impact of managed care on one training program: University of Florida at Gainesville. *Archived of Surgery, 130*(9), 929–930.

Cummings, N. A. (1995). Impact of managed care on employment and training: A primer for survival. *Professional Psychology: Research & Practice, 26*(1), 10–15.

Managed care has challenged many of professional psychology's training concepts and cherished attitudes. A number of changes that need to be made in professional education and training if psychology is to be a major player in the new health systems are discussed.

165

Dorsey, J. L. (1995). Last word: Witness to the revolution. *Hospitals & Health Networks, 69*(5), 58.

The origins of managed care in the 1960s are noted. Cost increases will probably level off and begin to drop by the end of the decade, as better-designed programs use vertically integrated systems funded by capitation to balance inpatient and outpatient services, and medical education emphasizes outpatient care and prevention.

Fischel, J. E., & Inkels, S. L. (1995). Managed care and medical education: Can these two entities interact? *Pediatrics, 96*(1), 171.

In a letter to the editor, Fischel and Inkels praise two discussions of managed care that were recently published in *Pediatrics* and set forth three considerations regarding managed care as it related to medical education.

Funding proposal shot in arm for HIV prevention in drug users. (1994). *AIDS Alert, 9*(8), 115–116.

A new $345 million treatment initiative included in President Clinton's 1995 federal budget proposal that could dramatically increase HIV prevention and drug treatment services for the estimated 2.7 million hard-core drug users is discussed. The funds would promote substance abuse treatment in managed care settings, among other things.

Hidden benefits of managed care. (1995). *Professional Psychology: Research & Practice, 26*(), 235–237.

Technical assistance and education, opportunities for socializing, the promotion of interdisciplinary collaboration, and free supervision are the four hidden benefits of managed care.

Marvin, J. A. (1995). Utilization of critical pathways in education. *Journal of Burn Care Rehabilitation, 16*(2, Pt. 2), 218.

Nahrwold, D. L. (1995). A hypothetical model for clinical education under managed care. *Archives of Surgery, 130*(9), 927–928.

Nelson, P. (1993). ANA to help develop managed care curriculum. *American Nursing, 25*(5), 25.

Page, L. (1995). New approaches to residency include managed care. *American Medical News, 38*(20), 25.

The medical education community is abuzz with plans to compile model managed care curricula, often through primary care initiatives, such as the Henry Ford Health System. Managed care says it needs physicians with a set of skills not traditionally taught in most residency programs or medical schools.

Sandrick, K. (1995). Training: Managed care 101. *Hospital Health Network, 69*(16), 46.

Schroeder, S. A. (1994). The latest forecast: Managed care collides with physician supply. *Journal of the American Medical Association, 272*(3), 239–240.

An editorial discusses the confluence of the dramatic growth of managed care and the impending oversupply of physician specialists.

Shea, C. (1995). Rx for student health? *Chronicle of Higher Education, 41*(30), A35–A36.

Some colleges and universities are turning to a managed care approach promoted by Collegiate Health Care for its campus infirmaries. The company has done well in rural colleges, but critics wonder if it will do as well in urban settings, where modern facilities are more readily available.

Sherer, J. L. (1993). Will college nursing education include managed care? *Hospital Health Network, 67*(13), 47.

Smith, I. (1994). Research moves out of the ivory tower. *REHAB Management, 7*(6), 62–64, 131–132.

The need to prove efficacy of treatment under managed care is outpacing academia's ability to produce that information.

Somerville, J. (1995). CMA study: High HMO administrative costs for Medicaid. *American Medical News, 38*(19), 9.

As states push Medicaid recipients toward managed care, the California Medical Association warns of high administrative costs in Medicaid health maintenance organizations (HMOs). The California Association of HMOs, however, says Medicaid HMOs offer services like patient education that hike administrative costs but also boost patient care.

Volger, J., & Ratliffe, C. E. (1993). Quality improvement and managed care as curriculum elements. *Nursing Education, 18*(3), 29–33.

MANAGED CARE RESOURCE ORGANIZATIONS

This information-only list of managed care resources includes such entities as publishers, policy groups, consultants, and professional associations. This list is not comprehensive, nor does it in any way represent the endorsement of the American Occupational Therapy Association, Inc.

American Association of Preferred Provider Organizations, 601 13th Street, N.W., Suite 370 South, Washington, DC 20005; 202-347-7600, 202-347-7601 (fax)

American Health Consultants, P.O. Box 71266, Chicago, IL 60691-9986; 800-688-2421, 800-850-1232 (fax)

American Health Information Management Association, 1919 Pennsylvania Avenue, N.W., Suite 300, Washington, DC 20006; 202-736-2155

American Managed Care and Review Association, 1200 19th Street, N.W., Suite 200, Washington, DC 20036; 202-728-0506, 202-728-0609 (fax)

American Medical Informatics Association, 4915 St. Elmo Avenue, Suite 302, Bethesda, MD 20814; 301-657-1291, 301-657-1296 (fax)

Blue Cross and Blue Shield Association, 676 North St. Clair Street, Chicago, IL 60611; 312-440-6000, 312-440-6609 (fax)

Center for Case Management, Inc., 6 Pleasant Street, South Natick, MA 01760; 508-651-2600, 508-655-0858 (fax)

Center for Health Policy Studies, c/o George Washington University, 2233 Wisconsin Avenue, N.W., Washington, DC 20007; 202-687-0880, 202-687-5229 (fax)

Executive Learning, Inc., 7101 Executive Center Drive, Suite 160, Brentwood, TN 37027; 800-929-7890 or 615-373-8483

Group Health Association of America, 1129 20th Street, N.W., Suite 600, Washington, DC 20036; 202-778-3200, 202-331-7487 (fax)

Health Insurance Association of America, 1025 Connecticut Avenue, N. W., Suite 1200, Washington, DC 20036-3998; 202-223-7780, 202-223-7889 (fax)

Health Outcomes Institute, 2001 Killebrew Drive, Suite 122, Bloomington, MN 55425; 612-858-9188, 612-858-9189 (fax)

Individual Case Management Association, 10809 Executive Center Drive, Suite 105, Little Rock, AR 72211; 501-954-7444, 501-227-8362 (fax)

Joint Commission on Accreditation of Healthcare Organizations, 1 Renaissance Boulevard, Oakbrook Terrace, IL 60181; 708-916-5000

Managed Care Information Center, 3100 Highway 138, Wall Township, NJ 07719-1442; 800-516-4343, 908-681-0490 (fax)

Managed Health Care Association, 1225 I Street, N.W., Suite 300, Washington, DC 20005; 202-371-8232, 202-842-0621 (fax)

Medical Group Management Association, 1275 Pennsylvania Avenue, N.W., Suite 503, Washington, DC 20004-2404; 202-659-0981, 202-466-7450 (fax)

National Committee for Quality Assurance, 1350 New York Avenue, N.W., Suite 700, Washington, DC 20005; 202-628-5788, 202-628-0344 (fax)

National Health Council, 1730 M Street, N.W., Washington, DC 20036; 202-785-3910

Utilization Review Group Accreditiation Commission, 1130 Connecticut Avenue, N.W., Suite 450, Washington, DC 20036; 202-296-9320

MANAGED CARE BOOKS

Boland, P. (Ed.). (1993). *Making managed healthcare work: A practical guide to strategies and solutions.* Gaithersburg, MD: Aspen Publishers.

Campbell, T., & McDevitt, D. D. (1994). *Health care antitrust: A manual for changing provider organizations.* New York: Thompson Publishing Group.

Giles, T. R. (1993). *Managed mental health care: A guide for practitioners, employers, and hospital administrators.* Boston: Allyn & Bacon.

Gingerich, B. S., & Ondeck, D. A. (Eds.). (1995). *Clinical pathways for the multidisciplinary home care team.* Gaithersburg, MD: Aspen Publishers.

Hendricks, R. L. (1993). *A model for national health care: The history of Kaiser Permanente.* New Brunswick, NJ: Rutgers University Press.

Howe, R. S. (Ed.). (1995). *Case management for health care professionals.* Chicago: Precept Press.

Introduction to clinical practice guidelines in health maintenance organizations. (1995). Washington, DC: Group Health Association of America.

Joint Commission on Accreditation of Healthcare Organizations. (1994). *Accreditation manual for health care networks. Vol. 2, Scoring.* Oakbrook Terrace, IL: JCAHO.

Joint Commission on Accreditation of Healthcare Organizations. (1994). *Accreditation manual for health care networks. Vol. 1, Standards.* Oakbrook Terrace, IL: JCAHO.

Kenkel, P. J. (1995). *Report card: What every health care provider needs to know about HEDIS and other performance measures.* Gaithersburg, MD: Aspen Publishers.

Krasner, M. I. (1995). *Monitoring Medicaid managed care: Developing an assessment and evaluation program.* New York: United Hospital Fund of New York.

Leyerle, B. (1994). *The private regulation of American health care.* Armonk, NY: M. E. Sharpe.

Linne, E. B. (1995). *Home care and managed care: Strategies for the future.* Chicago: American Hospital Association.

Managed health care: A resource guide. (1993). Tampa, FL: American College of Physician Executives.

Managed health care overview. (1994). Washington, DC: AMCRA Foundation.

National Conference on Managed Care Systems for Mothers and Young Children, April 13–14, 1993: Summary of conference proceedings. (1993). Portland, ME: National Academy for State Health Policy and Fox Health Policy Consultants.

Patient outcomes in managed care settings. (1993). Baltimore, MD: Williams & Wilkins.

Poynter, W. (1994). *The preferred provider's handbook: Building a successful private therapy practice in the managed care market.* New York: Brunner/Mazel.

Preparing for a changing healthcare marketplace: Lessons from the field. Washington, DC: Institute of Medicine.

Pyenson, B. (1995). *Calculated risk: A provider's guide to assessing and controlling the financial risk of managed care.* Chicago: American Hospital Pub.

Rowland, D. (1995). *Medicaid and managed care: Lessons from the literature: A report of the Kaiser Commission on the Future of Medicaid.* Washington, DC: Kaiser Commission.

Ruben, D. H. (Ed.). (1993). *Transitions: Handbook of managed care for inpatient to outpatient treatment.* Westport, CT: Praeger.

Satinsky, M. A. (1995). *An executive guide to case management strategies.* Chicago: American Hospital Pub.

Stuehler, G. (1995). *A collection of best practices of managed care organizations: The results of a survey by the Health Care Financing Administration, Office of Managed Care.* Washington, DC: U.S. GPO.

Winegar, N., & Bristline, J. L. (1994). *Marketing mental health services to managed care.* New York: Haworth Press.

Zander, K. S. (Ed.). (1995). *Managing outcomes through collaborative care: The application of caremapping and case management.* Chicago: American Hospital Association.

169

Index

173

174

Exclusive provider organizations (EPOs)
    explanation of, 14
    risk-sharing, 14, 18

F

Fee schedule, 21

Fee-for-service (FFS)
    contract issues regarding, 44
    discounted, 43, 49
    explanation of, 9, 21, 79
    health care spending due to, 2

Fieldwork
    example of program plan for, 115—121
    impact of managed care on, 109—111
    information and resources for, 122—124
    role of schools in facilitating success in, 113—114
    stress reduction in, 111—113

Fieldwork Data Form (American Occupational Therapy Association), 123

Fieldwork Evaluation for the Occupational Therapist (American Occupational Therapy Association), 124

Flexible health plans, 17

Flexible HMOs, 17

Foto, Mary, 1, 2

Foundations for medical care (FMCs), 15

Fraud. *See* Health care fraud/abuse

Fraud Alert on Joint Venture Arrangements (Office of the Inspector General)

Freedom-of-choice laws, 55—56

G

Gag clauses, 43, 59

Gatekeepers, 14

Grievance procedures, 59

Group Health Association (Washington, D.C.), 10

Group Health Cooperative of Puget Sound (Seattle), 10

Group Health Plan of Minneapolis, 10

Group insurance, 21

Group-model HMOs, 14, 78

The Guidelines for an Occupational Therapy Fieldwork Experience - Level I and Level II (American Occupational Therapy Association), 122

Health maintenance organizations (HMOs) (continued)
  group-model, 14, 78
  mixed-model, 16
  network-model, 16—17, 78
  open-ended, 17
  origins of, 10, 15
  payment methods of, 78, 79
  single-benefit, 18
  social, 18
  staff-model, 18, 78
Health Plan Employer Data and Information Set (HEDIS), 36—37
Health professional shortage areas (HPSAs), 22
Health-insuring organization (HIO). *See* Risk-sharing EPO
HMO swing-outs, 17
Hold harmless clauses, 40
Home health services
  clinical practice changes for, 72—73
  kickbacks in exchange for referral of reimbursable, 63—64
  organizational changes in, 72
Hybrid health plan. *See* Point-of-service (POS) plans
Hybrid HMOs, 17
Hybrid model plans, 17

I

Impairment, 93—94
Indemnification provisions, 40
Independent practice associations (IPAs)
  explanation of, 15, 22, 78
  origins of, 10, 15
Information Packet for Developing Student Affiliations (American Occupational Therapy Association), 122
Information reporting and disclosure requirements, 58
Information systems bibliography, 160
Insured, 22
Insurers, 22
Integrated delivery systems
  explanation of, 13
  fraud and abuse in, 62—64

J

Joint ventures, fraud and abuse in, 60—64

K

L

M

Managed care companies (continued)
      explanation of, 16, 19
Managed care organizations (MCOs)
      consumer protections and, 57—59
      contracts with, 39—49. *See also* Contracts
      function of, 1, 4, 6
      investigation of, 39—40, 46
      networks associated with, 49—54. *See also* Networks
      payment structure of, 43—44, 48, 77
      professional liability concerns and, 40—41, 46
      professional qualifications and performance requirements of, 41—42, 47
      provider participation regulation in, 55—57
      utilization management process of, 42—43, 47—48
Managed competition, 16
Managed indemnity plan (MIP), 16
Mandatory second opinions, 81
McCarthy, Diane, 105
Medicaid
      anti-kickback statute and, 60. *See also* Anti-kickback laws
      bibliography on, 147—148
      case managers for, 14
      explanation of, 23, 83
      managed care as element of, 4, 5, 83—84
      physician self-referral laws and, 61. *See also* Physician self-referral laws
      R/EPOs and, 18
      spending for, 3
Medical fee schedule, 23
Medicare
      anti-kickback statute and, 60. *See also* Anti-kickback laws
      assignment, 19
      bibliography on, 146
      carriers, 20
      explanation of, 23
      managed care as element of, 4—5, 81—82
      participating health care providers for, 24
      physician self-referral laws and, 61. *See also* Physician self-referral laws
      point-of-service option of, 83
      Prospective Payment System, 4
      spending for, 3
Medicare payment schedule, 23

182

Q

Quality assurance
    bibliography on, 154—156
    changes in practices regarding, 7
Quality control
    management techniques for, 81
    movement toward, 27

R

RBRVS (resource-based relative value scale), 24, 25
Regional fieldwork consultant (RFWC), 122
Reimbursement bibliography, 146—151
Relevant geographic market, 52
Relevant services market, 52
The Reliable Source, 124
Report cards
    background of, 35
    benefits and limitations of, 35—37
    conclusions regarding, 37—38
Risk management bibliography, 154—156
Risk pools, 43
Risk sharing
    under capitation, 80
    explanation of, 4
    in networks, 52
Risk withholds, 43
Risk-sharing EPO (R/EPO), 14, 18
RUC (RVS Update Committee), 25
Rule of reason analysis, 52
RVS (relative value scale), 25
RVU (relative value unit), 25

S

Safe harbors, 60, 61
San Joaquin County Foundation for Medical Care (Stockton, California), 10
Second opinions, mandatory, 81
Self-insurance
    explanation of, 25
    managed care contracts and groups with, 84